Home Accessibility
300 Tips for Making Life Easier

Shelley Peterman Schwarz

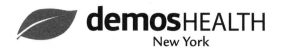

demosHEALTH

New York

Visit our website at www.demoshealth.com

ISBN: 978-1-936303-22-9
ebook ISBN: 978-1-617050-86-2

Acquisitions Editor: Noreen Henson
Compositor: Techset

Medical information provided by Demos Health, in the absence of a visit with a healthcare professional, must be considered as an educational service only. This book is not designed to replace a physician's independent judgment about the appropriateness or risks of a procedure of therapy for a given patient. Our purpose is to provide you with information that will help you make your own healthcare decisions.

The information and opinions provided here are believed to be accurate and sound, based on the best judgment available to the authors, editors, and publisher, but readers who fail to consult appropriate health authorities assume the risk of injuries. The publisher is not responsible for errors or omissions. The editors and publisher welcome any reader to report to the publisher any discrepancies or inaccuracies noticed.

Library of Congress Cataloging-in-Publication Data

CIP data is available from the Library of Congress.

Special discounts on bulk quantities of Demos Health books are available to corporations, professional associations, pharmaceutical companies, healthcare organizations, and other qualifying groups. For details, please contact:

Special Sales Department
Demos Medical Publishing
11 West 42nd Street, 15th Floor
New York, NY 10036
Phone: 800-532-8663 or 212-683-0072
Fax: 212-941-7842
E-mail: rsantana@demosmedpub.com

Printed in the United States of America by Hamilton Printing.
11 12 13 14/5 4 3 2 1

Home Accessibility

A Special Thank You

For over 9 years, I have had the best assistant and colleague to work with—Deborah Proctor. I know that it is only because of her many talents and skills that we have been able to tackle projects, large and small, and are now poised for even greater things in the future.

Deborah, you are an extraordinary researcher, writer, organizer, editor, idea generator, and marketing and overall project manager. As with so many things, I could not have written this book without you.

Thank you for all you do to make my life easier!

Contents

Foreword

Whether blindsided by an unforeseen injury or illness or slowly robbed of strength by the insidious ravages of old age, there will come a time for us all when we are rendered disabled and struggling or even unable to do for ourselves that which we previously took for granted. It is for these times that *Home Accessibility: 300 Tips for Making Life Easier* is of value; it will transform the reader from a victim to an empowered advocate.

My introduction to disability came at 4 years of age when my best friend's mother was diagnosed and bed-ridden with a progressive form of multiple sclerosis. At the time, I didn't really understand all the implications her disability had on her children, marriage, career, self-esteem, indeed her whole life. Over the years, I came to better appreciate how her disability shaped her environment—the homemade wooden ramp leading to the front door, the scooter she drove around the house, and the lift-equipped van she used to get around town—each of these adaptations allowed her to participate more with her family and rely less on others.

Despite my "enlightened" childhood, never did the concepts of *disability* and *accessibility* become more meaningful to me than three weeks before I was supposed to start medical school. In the blink of an eye, a roll-over car accident left me with a broken neck and rendered me quadriplegic. Robbed of my strength and independence, my dream of becoming a physician was threatened. I learned quickly that in order to get my life back on track I would not only have to undergo extensive rehabilitation therapies, but that adapting my environment was the key to achieving my dreams.

Twelve years later, I still call upon those early childhood lessons to not only maintain my independence, but also to empower my patients. Perhaps this is why I am so pleased to see this book come to market and why I am honored to write the foreword for this amazing book. May readers find within these pages the key to unlocking their potential and maximizing their independence.

Jonathan D. Myers, MD
Board Certified in Physical Medicine & Rehabilitation
Medical Director of Rehabilitation Services
St. Luke's Magic Valley Regional Medical Center
Twin Falls, ID

A Message From the Author

I have been very excited about writing *Home Accessibility: 300 Tips for Making Life Easier*. After living with multiple sclerosis (MS) for more than 30 years and using an Amigo™ three-wheeled scooter-style wheelchair for more than 25 years, I have learned a lot about making one's home safe and accessible. I have learned many of the tips through personal experience; others from friends, acquaintances, and the physical and occupational therapists who have helped me adjust and adapt to increasing disability.

In this book I have tried to present options for all budgets. Some of the suggestions I offer include no cost, using items you already have around your house. Others are of relatively low cost, less than $100. The information on Universal Design (UD) and more involved remodeling modifications is presented for those who have larger budgets or want to understand what makes a dwelling accessible. One of the primary resources I used to research this book was the Center for Universal Design (College of Design; North Carolina State University; Campus Box 8613; Raleigh, NC 27695-8613; Phone: 919-513-0825; www.design.ncsu.edu/cud). Their online guide *Residential, Rehabilitation, Remodeling, and Universal Design* is a valuable aid to anyone who needs to make modifications to accommodate physical limitations.

Whether you are recovering from surgery or an accident, living with a chronic illness or disability, or simply feeling the effects of your age (or know someone who is), my hope is that this book will help you find simple, cost-conscious solutions to keep you safe and independent in your home. And, in the process of reading this book, I hope you will discover tips, techniques, and timesavers that will make you say, "That's so simple! Why didn't I think of that?"

If you have a tip or product recommendation to share, I would love to learn about it. Visit www.MakingLifeEasier.com and submit your ideas or send me an email at Shelley@MakingLifeEasier.com.

Wishing you all the best.

Shelley
Follow Shelley on Twitter (ShelleyPSchwarz)
and Facebook (Shelley Peterman Schwarz)

Acknowledgments

I would like to thank the following people and organizations (in no specific order) who freely gave their time and knowledge educating me on specific needs of people with various disabilities different from my own. Without them this book would not have been possible.

Linda Lane and Pattie Dorn, Independent Living, Inc.; Dee Truhn and Belinda Richardson, Access to Independence; Susan Buzby and Regan Jacobsen, projecthome; Marshall Flax and Jean Kalscheur, Wisconsin Council of the Blind and Visually Impaired; Ellen McGinn, Meriter Hospital; Kelly Rehbeck, Center for Communication, Hearing, and Deafness—UniversaLink; Amy Wurf, Veteran's Administration; Larry Taff, TZ of Madison; Jim Klassy, Klassey, Inc.; Jeff Kichefski, Home Accessibility; Ruth Farrington, Marling Homeworks; Martine Davis, Indoor Environmental Testing Inc.; Rosemarie Rossetti, Universal Design Living Laboratory; and last but not least my wonderfully supportive friends and colleagues— Judy Ross, Carol Burns, Lisa Krosinski, and everyone else who has shared their tips and strategies for making life easier with me.

Who Needs This Book?

If you have picked up this book, chances are that you or someone in your life is struggling with some sort of limitation or disability. In fact, 70% of the population will have, at one time or another, difficulty climbing stairs or need to use a wheelchair. You are not alone in having to confront home accessibility issues.

This book has been written for anyone who is experiencing either a short-term disability such as after surgery or while healing a broken arm or leg, or a long-term chronic illness such as multiple sclerosis (MS), Parkinson's disease, or cancer. It is also for people who are challenged by sensory, vision, hearing, or tactile limitations; mental health issues including memory loss, dementia, and Alzheimer's disease; and for those who have had an accident, heart attack, stroke, or are getting older and find it more and more difficult to bend, reach, twist, and get up or down, in or out. This book provides support and information for the people who care about our safety, independence, and our quality of life.

You might be thinking, "Oh, I am just checking this out for my mother, father, aunt, uncle, grandparent . . . . However, you never know what life has in store for you. Remember—people with disabilities are the only minority group that anyone can join at any time!

I know because it happened to me. I was happy, healthy, married, and a mother of two young children, working my dream job as a teacher of the Deaf when odd little things began to bother me. I found myself tripping over nothing, no longer enjoying my favorite pastime, knitting, and my speed and ability to fingerspell to my students was "clumsy" and slowed. I was eventually diagnosed with the progressive form of multiple sclerosis (PPMS) and within a matter of a few years, I was in a wheelchair, with only minimal use of my left hand, unable to care for my most basic needs (let alone care for my young children), and dependent on others for nearly everything.

Over the years, I have learned how to cope with the loss of my abilities and have figured out ways to do many things, maintaining as much independence as possible. I have learned from others as well, observing and recording their tips and strategies. I began writing about what I learned and my articles were published in newspapers and magazines around the world. I even appeared on the Discovery Channel's popular *Home Matters* program, and have authored six *Tips for Making Life Easier*™ books. In this, my seventh book, I share the practical tips and strategies for making the home more accessible.

Creating an accessible home is something I think everyone should think about. After all, who would not enjoy wider hallways, open floor plans, and more light? If you are an empty nester and considering downsizing, think about choosing a home that you can live in, come what may. Limiting stairs, adding adjustable shower fixtures, and selecting easier-to-use faucets and door handles will provide you with a beautiful, livable home to be enjoyed now and well into the future. If you or a loved one are getting older and having difficulty maneuvering, what kinds of modifications can you do to make life easier and stay in your beloved home?

Our home is the center of our world; we raise our children, entertain friends, and often spend the majority of our life in our home. In this book, you will discover practical, relatively low-cost tips and strategies to make your life easier whether you have a chronic illness, a physical or sensory disability, or you or a loved one are struggling with the challenges that come with age. You will also find some things that, although pricier, may be well worth the investment if you wish to stay in your home for several years. If you and your family truly cannot afford these items and they are essential to your independence, often community agencies, independent living centers, support groups such as the National MS Society or Parkinson's Foundation, or even your faith community will help you with funding or know where to find it. And, along the way, I have sprinkled in a little inspiration and encouragement.

Included throughout the chapters of this book are products that I have found to make everyday tasks easier. Some are available in pharmacies or discount, building supply, and home improvement stores; others are unique and more difficult to find. A resources section at the end of each chapter will help you locate the items that are mentioned.

All contact information was accurate at the time this book was compiled, but keep in mind that a company's product offerings change from time to time. If you have difficulty locating a resource, vendor, or item listed in the resources section, search the Internet for current information. If you do not have an Internet connection, ask a family member or your librarian to help you search for what you need or send me an email at Shelley@MakingLifeEasier.com with your name and address.

I am not a physician, physical or occupational therapist, or rehabilitation specialist. I am someone who has faced the challenges of disability, learned along the way, and I share what I have learned with you here for your consideration. In addition to the tips I share here, I highly recommend and urge you to ask your doctor for a referral to a physical, occupational, or rehabilitation therapist for specific recommendations for what might make your life easier.

So to answer the question, "Who needs this book?" In a word, EVERYONE!

Home Is Where the Heart Is

ONE

Basic Concepts

LIVING WELL WITH LIMITATIONS

Being diagnosed with multiple sclerosis (MS) forced me to simplify my life. I was 32 years old and it was clear that life, as I knew it, had changed forever. As much as I wanted to deny it, I could not physically, mentally, or emotionally keep up the pace I had once demanded of myself. Over the years, I have realized that others with chronic illness and/or disabilities faced similar challenges. In fact, there are several overriding principles that everyone with a chronic medical condition or disability need to know:

- Take care of YOU first.
- Rejoice in what you can do and (try to) gracefully accept what you cannot.
- Take advantage of labor-saving devices and new technology.

I am reminded of a friend who had polio as a child. As she grew older, it became more and more difficult for her to breathe, yet she resisted using a ventilator thinking that it would limit her ability to go places outside of her home. In actuality, using the ventilator made it easier for her. She had more energy because she was not struggling to take every breath. Permitting herself to use this medical aid helped her to regain the ability to get out and about and do things that she had already given up because of her resistance. I was the same with regard to accepting having to use a wheelchair to get around. For both of us and others I know, as soon as we accepted our limitations and the help we needed, whether personal or mechanical, we were free to *live* our lives. Sometimes it is time to give in, although it is never time to give up.

WHEN HELPING A LOVED ONE

I encourage family and friends to be patient with the person you care about as he or she adjusts to his or her new reality. When someone faces the loss of abilities, it takes time to process the feelings and the fears. Most people do not like to admit that they can no longer do something; their sense of who they are is affected. They may feel frustrated, angry, and less of a person, and they often take those feelings out on those they love the most. One needs to understand that all these emotions are a normal, natural part of the grieving process. You and your loved one are grieving the loss of the person they once knew, and facing an unknown future is scary. In time, healing begins, and acceptance begins to replace anger and frustration.

If you feel that the person you care about is depressed or "stuck" in denial or anger it is important to communicate that to his or her doctor. Perhaps you should offer to accompany your friend or family member to the doctor's office. Often, medications and/or talk therapy can help one transition to a more accepting attitude.

Another option might be to enlist the counsel of a trusted friend or clergy person to speak with your loved one about his or her new reality and assure him or her that giving in does not make him or her any less loved.

These last two suggestions are especially important if one's family does not live in the same town. An extra pair of eyes and ears can alert you to changes that may need your attention.

ATTITUDES ARE CONTAGIOUS

As the children's song says, "Look on the sunny side, always on the sunny side . . . ." Cry over your loss if you need to, but then begin to look for the light, the things that really matter, and the relationships you have with those around you.

Laugh about the frustrations; they will not go away, but you will feel better. Remember it takes fewer muscles to smile than to frown. Besides, others will enjoy being around you more and your life will open up simply because you find humor even in difficult situations.

PRINCIPLES FOR LIVING WELL WITH A CHRONIC ILLNESS OR DISABILITY

Before I get into specific home accessibility tips, I would like to share some of the most basic lessons for living well regardless of your temporary or permanent situation. Life is all about choices and I am convinced that if you or your loved one chooses to follow these basic principles you will feel better, have more control, and get more enjoyment out of your life.

- **Keep balance in your life.** Prioritize, eliminate, consolidate, and streamline activities in all aspects of your life.

- **Take care of yourself.** Be sensible about how you spend your time and energy. Do the things that are most important to you and to your family. Try to eliminate unnecessary or difficult tasks. Give yourself permission to rest. Make compromises and remove the words "I should" from your vocabulary.

- **Pace your activities.** Try to break an activity down into a series of smaller tasks. Rest before you become exhausted and, if required, enlist the help of others.

- **Eat a healthy diet.** Do not skip meals. Carry trail mix, nuts, and/or fresh fruits with you. Eat a healthy snack and avoid the temptation to grab a candy bar with hollow calories and little nutritional value.

- **Arrange your home for your convenience.** Sometimes this means putting handrails or grab bars in strategic locations to help you walk from room to room or placing a chair halfway down a long hallway so that you can stop to rest. Sometimes it means purchasing duplicate cleaning supplies for both upstairs and downstairs, or kitchen, bathroom, and laundry room, so that you do not have to spend excess energy going back and forth. Only you know what this means for you.

- **Ask for help when you need it.** Take advantage of products, services, and people that are available. When you need something or someone to help you, do not look at it as giving in, but instead look at it as making intelligent decisions that will make your life easier and safer. Besides, asking for help gives others the pleasure of doing a good deed. (You know how good you feel when you do something for someone else.)

- **Use technology.** New technology is created everyday that may make it easier for you to do what you want to do. Remote controlled devices and cordless phones save steps. Speaker phones, voice mail, and wireless intercoms can be used to save time and energy. Computers are good for keeping records, keeping a journal, and writing letters. A smartphone can keep you connected and synchronizes with your computer to help you keep track of people, appointments, and your schedule all in one place. An Internet connection can expand your horizons, whether doing research on your condition or providing opportunities to communicate with others. Keep abreast of technological changes and make full use of every option helpful to you. (Find more information in Chapter 9—The Accessible Office: Putting Technology to Work for You.)

- **Use labor-saving devices.** There are many labor-saving devices available to make almost any task easier. For example, reachers come in various lengths, weights, and means of operation. Find the styles that work for you in various situations (reaching cans on a shelf, picking something up off the floor, etc.). Timers, magnifiers, organizers, special telephones, and light switch extenders are just a few of the many products that may make everyday tasks easier for you to accomplish.

- **Learn all that you can about your condition.** Research books at the library and online sources for information on your condition. There are also agencies and organizations that can help you meet your personal life challenges. Visit websites such as www.Sharecare. com to find answers to your health-related questions by health experts—neurologists, physiatrists, orthopedists, rheumatologists, radiologists, nurses, occupational, physical, and speech therapists, dietitians, and more.

- **Consider joining a support group.** You are not alone! There are others who have walked a similar path before you. Learn from them by attending a support group that focuses on your specific limitation or disability. To find an agency or support group near you, ask your doctor or get a list of agencies from your local library or United Way office. You might also contact a local hospital or clinic to see if they offer coping-type support groups for people with chronic illness or those who are going through life-altering changes. Look for websites such as www.PatientsLikeMe.com where you will find an online community of people with various disabilities sharing support and encouragement.

- **Enlist the aid of a physical, occupational, or rehabilitation therapist.** Ask your doctor or hospital rehabilitation department about a referral to an occupational or physical therapist and you will learn about which assistive products would be most helpful to you. Be honest about your abilities and goals so that the assessment and recommendations they make will offer the most benefit for you.

- **Contact your local independent living center (ILC).** Every community in the United States is part of a national network of more than 500 community-based, nonprofit ILCs that serve people of all ages and disabilities and their families. ILCs provide information and referral to community services, offer advocacy training and peer support groups, and teach independent living skills. The following are a few examples of their many services:
  - Assist you in finding out about disability services in your community.
  - Connect you with others to advocate for changes in the laws or rules.
  - Help you hire and manage personal care attendants.
  - Put you in contact with people who have faced challenges similar to that of your own.

Most centers have a lending library of adaptive gadgets and devices you may try for a while at no cost. When you find what works for you, they can use their vast computer database of companies and manufacturers that make these products and help you order what you need.

Your local library, hospital, senior center, United Way office, or your state, county, Catholic, Lutheran, or Jewish social services agency should be able to assist you in finding the nearest ILC. For a national directory of ILCs, contact the National Council on Independent Living. Additional resources are found at the end of the chapters.

For "15 Tips for Staying Independent" visit my website, www. MakingLifeEasier.com. Look for more tips, products, coping strategies, and inspiration for living life well despite limitations.

RESOURCES

National Council on Independent Living
1710 Rhode Island Avenue NW
Fifth Floor
Washington, DC 20036
Phone: 202-207-0334
Toll free: 877-525-3400
TTY: 202-207-0340

Meeting Life's Challenges, LLC
The home of Tips for Making Life Easier
9042 Aspen Grove Lane
Madison, WI 53717
Phone: 608-824-0402
www.MeetingLifesChallenges.com
www.MakingLifeEasier.com

Your Home Is Your Castle

TWO

Home Adaptations

When my husband Dave and I were looking to buy our first home we only looked at two-story houses. Both of us had been raised in two-story houses. In fact, we put in a bid on a split-foyer house, where, when you enter, you either have to go upstairs or downstairs to get to the living space. We were only $500 shy of what the seller was asking and we felt we could not go up any higher than our offer.

A few weeks later, with nothing to do on a cold, dreary, and windy Sunday in March, we went to see a ranch-style house that was for sale by the owner. As we walked out Dave asked, "What do you think?" I responded, "It's okay, but it's not my dream house."

Three weeks later I had the most vivid dream. A voice told me to buy the ranch-style house. I woke up the next morning and told Dave that we were supposed to buy that house, and by dinner we had an accepted offer.

Mind you, at the time we were house hunting I was perfectly healthy and had no idea that 6 years later I would be diagnosed with MS, and that 4 years after I would need a wheelchair. We lived in that ranch house for 26 years. Had we purchased a two-story house like we had planned, we would have had to move because of my special needs.

Even though our ranch-style house was more accessible than most of the homes in my neighborhood, our home still had "issues" that created barriers for me. For example, the washer and dryer were down in the basement, the tub and shower were not accessible, there were three steps from the garage into the house, and the front door had two steps, which meant that in an emergency I could not get out of the house.

Our first remodeling project was 2 years after my diagnosis, when we brought the laundry facilities up to the first floor. We also added railings to both sides of the stairway from the garage into the house. A few years later, we added on to our bedroom making room for an electric bed for me. We also wired a special switch box so that I could operate the lights and overhead fan from the bed, and created an accessible bathroom with a raised toilet, open area under the sink, and a roll-in shower.

Although these projects were costly, it allowed us to stay in our home. I know that making some homes accessible would be nearly impossible or cost prohibitive, but I also know that sometimes simple little tweaks can create a livable situation—not perfect but acceptable.

Although some home modifications included in this book may be more costly than others, this book is primarily about affordable adaptations that you can make to your home to make life easier. In the chapters that follow, you will find hundreds of tips for adaptations you may be able to easily make yourself. However, I would be remiss if I did not address what to do or who to call when you need help or, even more importantly, without giving you the basic parameters such as how much space you need to turn a wheelchair, the best location for light switches and faucets, or the basics of "universal design."

This chapter sets the stage for determining your home's accessibility by helping you define what you need and who to call. Adaptations for those who are Deaf, hard of hearing, have low vision, blind, and other disabilities not involving mobility will be addressed in each chapter of Section III: The Accessible Home: Room by Room.

RETROFITTING, REMODELING, AND CUSTOM DESIGN

Studies by AARP show that 75% of people aged 45 and older and 88% to 90% of older adults aged 65 and older wish to stay in their own home for as long as possible. This is called "aging in place."

Yet, most homes that our older loved ones live in do not have the wider doors and hallways, accessibility features, or space in the bathroom, kitchen, and bedroom to make this possible. This means that you either need to make adaptations yourself as you or a loved one needs them, hire a professional to retrofit your home as much as possible to meet your needs within the confines of the original home, remodel your home by perhaps changing walls, bumping out space, or adding rooms, or if you are younger—in your 50s or 60s—buying or building your dream home; the one you intend to live in for life. In each case there are specific parameters that you will want to be familiar with so you can determine what you can do yourself, when to hire a professional and, perhaps more importantly, so you can ask intelligent questions and avoid costly mistakes.

KNOW WHAT YOU NEED AND GET HELP FINDING ANSWERS

One of the accessibility problems in our house was the sunken living room. You saw it the minute you walked in the front door. It was lovely and dramatic. When I was unable to walk any longer and needed my three-wheeled Amigo® scooter to get around the house, I just did not go into the living room. On special occasions, my husband Dave would carry me into the room and put me in the rocker/recliner where I stayed until he carried me back to my Amigo.

In our minds it was impossible to ramp the living room without losing the charm and unique design feature. When we invited a decorator over to help us choose new carpet and furniture, he thought it was awful that I could not enjoy the entire house and quickly came up with a plan to ramp the living room that was absolutely brilliant; something we had never thought of.

Whether you have your own specific ideas on what you need and want, or you feel totally lost and overwhelmed with even the smallest project, here are some points to get you started.

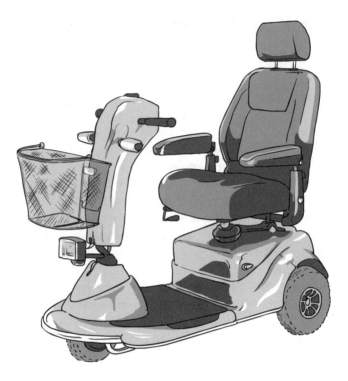

BASIC QUESTIONS AND ANSWERS

How much space do you need to back up and turn around when you are in a wheelchair?

Answer: The standard wheelchair needs a minimum of 5 feet (**60″** × **60″**) to turn around. Actually, a space longer than wider (63″ × 56″ is often preferable, especially in the kitchen and bathroom). This holds true for walkers too.

How wide do doorways need to be to keep from scraping my knuckles?

Answer: For a wheelchair or a person on a walker to get through without scraping knuckles, doorways need to be a minimum of 32 inches, but preferably 36 inches wide.

How big does the space in front of a door need to be, so that you can easily open it?

Answer: The turning radius of your wheelchair (see above), plus 18 to 24 inches of clearance on the side of the door that opens (so that you can get around it).

Where do things need to be located so you can reach them from your wheelchair?

Answer: The average person can reach a maximum of 48 inches to the front and 54 inches to the side, no higher than 52 to 60 inches and no lower than 9 inches on the side or 12 inches in front. Countertops should be 27 to 32 inches high depending on work to be done there. *Note*: If you are taller, your range of reach will be more, if you are shorter, your range of reach will be less. Adjust accordingly.

You will find more information on dimensions in the Accessibility Guidelines sidebars at the beginning of most chapters.

WHEN TO HIRE A PROFESSIONAL

There are many simple modifications that you can do yourself but when it comes to bathrooms, kitchens, bigger projects, or safety issues, it is usually better to hire a professional who is experienced in aging in place, universal design, or both. The building industry, which includes architects, builders, interior designers, and other building specialists, and the remodeling industry both offer aging in place certification. Though, as I write this, certification is relatively new and thus certified aging in place specialists (CAPS) are rare. Thankfully certification is becoming more and more of an industry standard all the time.

The cost of retrofitting a bathroom or kitchen to make it more accessible can easily exceed $25,000, a figure that is much higher than building for the future right from the start. If you are considering building or adding on to a home, talk with your builder or architect about using universal design principals. It may cost a little more up front, but it will be less expensive to build it with the future in mind than to have to retrofit or remodel later. And homes built with universal design elements often maintain a higher resale value over the life of the home.

Whether you choose to retrofit an existing space, remodel your current home, or build for the future, before hiring a professional, be sure to ask about CAPS certification or about their specific knowledge and experience with aging in place or universal design principles. If they look at you like you are speaking a foreign language or try to excuse those terms as being unnecessary, keep looking. If they say they have experience, check out their references.

Be sure to interview previous clients who have had accessibility modifications completed. The last thing you want is to spend a lot of time and money to make your home more accessible and find out afterward that it is not much better than it was before. Believe me, this has happened.

WHERE TO FIND ADVICE

In researching this section I was amazed at how much information is available on how to make your home more accessible.

- Local area councils on aging are a great resource for older adults. Look in your phone book or ask your librarian to help you locate a council near you.
- AARP has conducted studies and webinars educating the public and building industry on how to create a "home for life" that encourages living independently. It offers a series of housing and mobility publications. Check out the Home Improvement section at www.AARP.org.
- Architecture schools that teach universal design (learn more about universal design in Chapter 3) offer a wealth of information online and in free or low-cost publications.
- Home assessment checklists at AARP and commercial websites such as www.AdaptMy.com ask a series of questions to help you determine your accessibility needs.

RESOURCES

The National Association of the Remodeling Industry (NARI) trains remodeling contractors on how to remodel houses to help those with limitations due to aging or disabilities remain independent and stay in their homes longer and more safely. If you need help making your home more accessible, contact the NARI chapter in your area and ask for referrals to remodeling contractors who are certified or specialize in aging in place. To find a chapter near you, visit the national NARI website at www.NARI.org.

The National Association of Home Builders (NAHB) provides a state-by-state directory of building professionals that will help you find a Certified Aging in Place Specialist in your area. If you do not

have access to the Internet, contact your local library to locate the office near you or contact National Association of Home Builders (NAHB)
201 15th Street NW
Washington, DC 20005
Phone: 202-266-8200
Toll free: 800-368-5242
www.NAHB.com

Aging in Place Professionals is an organization who's mission is to help people to safely and creatively remain in their home of choice for as long as confidently possible. A wide array of professionals are represented—builders, remodelers, architects, interior designers, and related professionals—and they are a wealth of information. Check out their online home tour videos demonstrating universal design principles in an actual home.
Phone: 626-799-5900
www.aipathome.com

PRODUCT

Amigo® Scooter
Amigo Mobility International, Inc.
6693 Dixie Highway
Bridgeport, MI 48722
Phone: 800-MY-AMIGO (800-692-6446)
www.MyAmigo.com

THREE

Accessibility, Visit-ability, and Universal Design

When you depend on a mobility device like a walker, wheelchair, or scooter, you quickly learn that "accessibility" means different things to different people. Even when you have the most accessible apartment or condo, if snow is piled in the wheelchair-accessible parking space and "curb cut," access to your home is denied.

Snow is a temporary obstacle. The snow will melt or it will be shoveled into a pile of snow in another area. However, stairs, surface changes, poorly lit rooms, heavy doors, noisy rooms, and cluttered spaces are only a few of the household barriers that can pose challenges for us.

Wouldn't it be nice if homes were designed without any barriers at all?

Soon you may see just that. Rising out of the civil rights movement of the 1960s, growing and maturing over several decades, through the Americans with Disabilities Act of 1990 and 2010 and the Fair Housing Act of 1998, and fueled by baby boomers wishing to age gracefully in their own homes, three philosophies have emerged encouraging the design of products and features in homes and buildings that allow people of *all* abilities to live their lives unimpeded by physical barriers. Here's a brief explanation of the current terminology.

ACCESSIBILITY

Accessibility focuses on disability. Features are added to a living space to accommodate a particular limitation. A toilet seat may be raised, a faucet changed, grab bars installed in the bathroom, doors removed to make the doorway wide enough for a wheelchair to pass, ramps, portable or permanent lifts, strobe light alerts, and tactile or Braille markers are all examples of accessibility features. Often recommendations are made by a physical or occupational therapist when someone loses their ability to lift, reach, grasp, bend, walk, see, hear, and so on due to advancing age or after a debilitating illness or injury.

VISIT-ABILITY

Visit-ability means making every house—not just special houses for people with disabilities—accessible to all. The concept is that everyone should be able to visit their friends and neighbors, regardless of ability, without barriers. Visit-ability advocates feel that every house should have:

- One exterior door with a step-free entrance
- All interior doors on the entry level should be at least 32 (preferably 36) inches wide to allow wheelchair access
- An accessible bathroom on the entry level

Visit-ability concentrates on access for people with physical disabilities that affect mobility, primarily those who use wheelchairs (though those with other disabilities may benefit as well). If every home were built or remodeled to include just these three features, every home would be visit-able by everyone. Add a bedroom on the first floor and no one should have to move from their home simply because of a disability.

UNIVERSAL DESIGN

Universal design is the most all-encompassing philosophy. It asks the question, "How do you design a space that functions equally well for *all* users?" The goal is a home that allows everyone, not just people with disabilities, easy access and livability by incorporating accessibility features into the overall design of the structure in a tasteful and barely perceivable way. The design of the products and living environments are to be usable by all people, to the greatest extent possible, without the need for adaptation or specialized design.

This means wider doors and hallways to allow greater ease of movement whether used by a mother carrying a child and a bag of groceries or someone using a walker; raised dishwashers and front-loading washers and dryers with front controls that are easier to load and unload from both a standing and seated position; higher kick plates under cabinets and open spaces under sinks that give a sleek look while allowing someone in a wheelchair the ability to use them; contrasting counters and floors that aid people with visual disabilities to "see" the edges; raised electric outlets that are safer for children and reduce the need for adults to bend over; lowered rocker-style light switches that even a child can operate; pot-filling faucets at the stove so that you do not have to carry heavy pots across the kitchen; nonslip flooring that is safer for all sorts of feet; more natural light for better visibility; and walk-in showers with multiple shower heads that are suitable for all regardless of height.

Wouldn't you say that all these features would make your home a nicer place in which to live regardless of whether you had a disability or not?

It is conservatively estimated that up to 60% of all new houses will, over the lifetime of the home, be occupied by a resident with severe, long-term mobility impairment (Smith et al., 2008). The point of my sharing a summary of these philosophies with you is to encourage those of you who are reading this book who may be remodeling or building or purchasing a home to consider incorporating universal design features throughout. That way, when (not if) the time comes that you need more room to get around, a more accessible kitchen or bathroom, more light to see, or fewer steps to climb you will already have them and you can gracefully "age in place" and not have to move because of physical limitations.

Numerous universal design principles are mentioned throughout this book. For more information on design features that you can live with for a lifetime, see the Resources section accompanying this chapter.

RESOURCES

Accessibility, Visit-ability, and Universal Design

Concrete Change
600 Dancing Fox Road
Decatur, GA 30032
Phone: 404-378-7455
www.concretechange.org

The Center for Universal Design
Universal Design Imitative: CUD | RED Lab
College of Design
North Carolina State University
Campus Box 8613
Raleigh, NC 27695-8613
www.design.ncsu.edu/cud

The Center for Inclusive Design and Environmental Access (IDEA)
378 Hayes Hall, School of Architecture and Planning
3435 Main Street
University at Buffalo
Buffalo, NY 14214-3087
Phone: 716-829-5902
www.ap.buffalo.edu/idea

National Resource Center on Supportive Housing and Home Modification
National and international resources, directory of home modification programs, library, news, links to government and private web sites on aging resources and services
Andrus Gerontology Center
University of Southern California
3715 McClintock Ave
Los Angeles, CA 90089-0191
Phone: 213-740-1364
www.homemods.org

Universal Design Demonstration Homes and Displays

Eskaton Livable Design National Demonstration Home
1621 Eskaton Loop
Roseville, CA 95747

Phone: 916-334-1072
Toll free: 888-933-6646
www.demohome.org

Freedom House
The Green Mountain Ranch
1331 Green Mountain Drive
Livermore, CO 80536
Phone: 970-484-4182
Video: http://www.aipathome.com/showcases/aip-homes-
communities/green-mountain-ranch/

The LiveAbility House
Kansas State University
Adult Development and Aging
343 Justin Hall
Manhattan, KS 66506
Phone: 785-532-5773
www.aging.ksu.edu
Watch the virtual home tour at:
http://www.thynkalittle.com/index.php?option=com_content&
view=article&id=51&Itemid=67

Show House
The Universal Design Alliance
3651-E Peachtree Parkway, Suite 311
Suwanee, GA 30024
Phone: 770-667-4591
www.universaldesign.org

Sunset Pines Resort
Fully accessible cabins
W9210 Rock Creek Road
Willard, WI 54493
Phone: 715-267-6989
www.sunsetpinesresort.com

Universal Design Living Laboratory
Columbus, OH
Phone: 614-471-6100
www.UDLL.com

WelcomeHOME Bed and Breakfast
4260 W. Hawthorne Drive
West Bend, WI 53090
Phone: 262-675-2525
WelcomeHOME@hnet.net

A Few Books

Accessible Home Design: Architectural Solutions for the Wheelchair User
Paralyzed Veterans of America Press, 2006
Toll free: 888-860-7244
Also available on Amazon.com

Universal Design Specifications and Home Plans
Universal Design Imitative: CUD | RED Lab, 2000
College of Design
North Carolina State University
Campus Box 8613
Raleigh, NC 27695-8613
www.design.ncsu.edu/cud

Websites

AARP
601 E Street, NW
Washington, DC 20049
Toll free: 888-OUR-AARP (888-687-2277)
Toll free TTY: 877-434-7589
Toll free Spanish: 877-627-3350
www.aarp.org
Search CAPS (Certified Aging in Place Specialists) and Universal
Design Webinar at:
http://www.aarp.org/home-garden/home-improvement
info-09-2010/home_design_webinar.html

Ability Awareness
Volunteers with disabilities build homes for people with disabilities
PO Box 10878
Costa Mesa, CA 92627
Phone: 949-854-8700
www.AbilityAwareness.org

Aging in Place Professionals
Phone: 626-799-5900
www.aipathome.com

Living with Universal Design—checklist
The Prince William Area Agency on Aging
5 County Complex Court, Suite 240
Woodbridge, VA 22192
Phone: 703-792-6400
See the home checklist at http://www.pwcgov.org/docLibrary/PDF/003529.pdf

Universal Designers and Consultants
For ideas, view the case studies and multi-media gallery at:
www.UniversalDesign.com

REFERENCE

Smith, S. K., Rayer, S., & Smith, E. A. (2008). Aging and disability: Implications for the housing industry and housing policy in the United States. *Journal of the American Planning Association, 74*(3), 289–306.

The Accessible Home:
Room by Room

FOUR

Coming In, Going Out

Accessibility in your home starts at your front door. Let's face it—if you cannot easily get in or out of the house, you are not going to get very far. I remember when I started using my little three-wheeled Amigo scooter because I could no longer walk from one end of our ranch-style house to the other. While I could still walk a few feet and maneuver a step or two, I knew it wouldn't be long before those limited abilities would make it impossible for me to get in or out of my house independently.

I suggested to my husband Dave that it might be a good idea to add a ramp to the front door. So, one beautiful spring day he and a friend decided to build the ramp. They were so excited to take on this project! It took them two days to plan, measure, purchase the materials, and construct it. From inside the house, I could hear them cutting, hammering and, finally, admiring their handiwork.

Accessibility Guidelines

To accommodate a wheelchair, scooter, or walker:

- *Pathways and ramps should be 4 feet wide.*
- *Sidewalk slopes or ramps should rise no more than 1 inch for every 12 inches in length; a 1 to 20 ratio is more manageable when pushing or propelling a manual wheelchair.*
- *Add a flat, 5-foot-long rest area to ramps and slopes at least every 30 inches in rise and at every 90° corner.*
- *Railings should be 1.5 inches in diameter and 1.5 inches from any wall or other structures.*
- *Railings should be built to support 250 pounds at any point along their length.*
- *For someone in a wheelchair to open a door, they will need 18 to 24 inches of clear space on the side where the door opens.*
- *You will need a space 15 to 16 feet wide and 7 to 8 feet high to accommodate an accessible van.*

When the ramp was finished they called me to try it out. As soon as they opened the front door I could see a very steep ramp that went directly from the threshold of the door to the sidewalk below. There was no landing on which I could exit the door, close it behind me, and drive slowly down the ramp. Oops! We all looked at each other and started laughing. This was definitely a case of "I guess we should have read the directions before we started."

Building to accommodate physical and sensory limitations takes some planning. To help get you started I offer the following ideas.

SIDEWALKS AND PATHS

Often, the most significant barrier in getting into and out of the home for people with mobility or sensory limitations is the entranceway itself. Many people think that a ramp is the only solution and hate the idea of advertising their disability by adding one. But ramps are not the only way to make an entrance accessible.

Sometimes a little creative landscaping can provide a level or slightly sloped path from the sidewalk or driveway to the house. "Ramping" can be achieved by building up the grade and adding landscaping to enhance a new accessible walkway. A curved walkway winding past plantings could be a lovely way to enter your home.

1. **Ask a landscaper for ideas on creating an accessible entryway.** When you do, keep the following guidelines in mind:

   - **Pathways should be 4 feet wide** to allow easy maneuvering of a wheelchair or walker; that width also allows two people to walk side-by-side comfortably.
   - **If possible, slopes should be limited to a 1-inch rise for every 20 inches in length;** though ADA requirements for ramps only require a 1 to 12 ratio, this is too steep for pushing or propelling a manual wheelchair—or a walker—any distance, especially if you do not have handrails on both sides to help you.
   - **Flat rest areas, at least 5 feet long, should be provided for every 3 feet of continuous rise.** Place a raised garden bed with a bench off to the side of the walk for those who may need to sit down and rest a moment.
   - **Build in some handrails along the way,** if not the entire length of the sloped area (recommended), then at corners and key

locations. Make them decorative or part of flower boxes and plantings and they will blend into the overall setting.

2. **Use contrasting railings and plantings, even colored cement,** to help those with poor vision more easily "see" where the sidewalk leads.

3. **Texture concrete surfaces.** When adding new walkways, brush the wet cement with a broom while still wet before setting to give the walk some grip under foot. For an existing sidewalk, there are nonslip coatings that can be applied to ramps and walkways; ask about these at your local home improvement store.

4. **Extend sidewalks to the door** ending with a large (a minimum 5 feet square), flat landing area (no step) in front of the door.

ENTRYWAYS

Once you get to the door is there a high threshold that is hard to get over? Anything higher than one-half inch is a safety hazard to someone in a wheelchair or who has difficulty seeing or walking. When building or remodeling, insist on a barrier-free entry on at least one door (preferably two for the sake of safety). If you are retrofitting an existing home, here are a few ideas to help you get through the door.

5. **Lower your threshold.** If the threshold is wood, a quick fix is to sand down the edges on each side (interior and exterior) to create a smooth hump that is easier to slide or roll over. If you need a longer lead way to get over a particularly high threshold, try making a wedge out of a standard piece of lumber (1×2 inches to 1×6 inches will likely work best) and affix it to the edge of your current door threshold. Ask at the lumber yard if they might cut and sand it down for you.

6. **Invest in a portable threshold.** If sanding your door threshold is not possible due to materials, door design, or because you rent, there is a reasonably low-cost solution—a portable threshold ramp that sits over the existing one. Made of lightweight but sturdy aluminum, the ramp extends the width of the threshold, making a gentler transition into the house. The advantage of this ramp is that you can fold it up and take it with you if you move or when visiting the homes of friends and family whose doorways may provide a challenge.

7. **Purchase a threshold ramp to get over small steps.** If you only
   have one small step (2–4 inches) to maneuver, there are a
   variety of threshold ramps that will give you the lift you need.
   To get an idea of what is available, go to www.discountramps.
   com. If you prefer to build your own, a height of 2 to 4 inches
   will require a length of 24 to 48 inches; it should be sturdy
   enough to support 400 pounds or more. Ask your Independent
   Living Center (ILC) for recommendations or about trying one
   that might be in their lending library.

8. **Paint thresholds, door frames, and knobs in a color that contrasts with the door and siding,** and mark any changes in height
   with high-contrast paint. This will help those with visual limitations "see" the difference and easily identify doors and hazards.

RAMPS AND RAILINGS

Ramps

If you use a wheelchair or scooter, or even a walker, ramps are much
easier to negotiate than stairs. Ramps can be as lovely as a nice deck,
built to enhance the look of your home or as utilitarian and portable
as modular aluminum (often a better choice if the home is not your
own). Aluminum ramps can be expensive, ranging up to $5,000. If
you need one, community agencies will often help you find an affordable way to obtain one. For assistance, start by calling your local Independent Living Center (ILC) or United Way (just dial 211) and tell
them what you need; they will give you referrals to appropriate
local agencies.

You might also ask your faith community to help defray expenses.
Contact your local NARI or NAHB for a referral to a building contractor that specializes in accessible remodeling and ask for a
quote. Contact information for both organizations is included in
the Resource section of Section II, Chapter 2.

9. **Keep accessibility guidelines in mind** when deciding if and what
   kind of ramp is best for you.

   • **Ramps work best for heights up to 30 inches;** over that you will
     most likely need a vertical lift or elevator.

- **The slope or rise should be no more than 1 inch for every 12 inches in length.** As noted earlier, this ratio is quite steep, especially for someone in a manual wheelchair or walker. A 1-inch rise for every 20 inches is easier to maneuver, but of course this makes the ramp longer.
- **Guard against the mobility device slipping off the ramp** by adding a 4-inch guard along the bottom edge along the entire length of the ramp.
- **The ramp should be 48 inches wide** with a minimum of 42 inches of clear space between railings on both sides.
- **Rest and/or turning areas at least 5 feet long need to be provided**
  - 3 feet of rise in elevation
  - 30 feet in unbroken length
  - at every 90-degree turn AND
  - in front of the entry door

10. **Make sure your ramp has a nonslip surface** by adding:

    - 1 pound silica sand/gallon of paint (be sure to stir often); or sprinkle the sand on top of wet paint as you go.
    - Rolled roofing paper tacked down securely to provide traction.
    - Battens, which are thin strips of wood that stop wheels from rolling backward, you will have to power your wheelchair over.

11. **Keep required maintenance in mind.** The materials you use to build the ramp must allow easy leaf, ice, and snow removal without deteriorating too quickly. Wooden ramps should be constructed of preservative-treated lumber, and will require regular painting and staining. Be sure to slope all flat areas one-eighth of an inch to one side for drainage.

Note: As always, "Try before you buy." Your local ILC may have samples of aluminum ramps in their loan closet. Visit senior centers to see what they have installed and ask the people there what they chose and why, or ask builders and contractors for referrals to accessible homes they have worked on and ask the owners what worked for them. You can find free, do-it-yourself ramp plans at www.handiramp.com.

Railings

12. **Railings should be 1.5 inches in diameter with a 1.5-inch clearance** between the inside of the railing and any wall or support.

Anything more than 1.5 inches becomes a hazard as an arm might slip through and get caught.

13. **Extend railings at least 1 foot beyond the end of any ramp** (top and bottom) to give someone in a wheelchair enough length to pull the chair ahead to the level space. It is a good idea to add a support pole at this spot for stability and to keep someone from running into the extra length of railing.

14. **Railings should be built to support a force of 250 pounds at any point.**

Lifts

If the entry to your home is particularly high, and a long ramp impractical, a vertical lift might be the solution. The cost of lifts, including a concrete slab, electrical power, and related remodeling expenses can range between $5,000 and $15,000. Social service agencies (Catholic, Jewish, or Lutheran Social Services, United Way, and others in your community) may be able to help you apply for grants and low-interest loans. Your faith community might also help you defray the cost. Remember, if you need the lift to get out of your house to go to work, your state vocational rehabilitation agency may also help cover the cost.

15. **Vertical platform lifts** work like an elevator to raise a wheelchair or scooter, along with a companion, smoothly and effortlessly straight up and down from driveway or entry path to entryway, patio, or porch. Most will rise about 4.5 feet but some will go as high as 14 feet, enough to reach the second floor. Taking up less than 30 square feet of space, a vertical platform wheelchair lift can avoid the space problems of long ramps. A lift, powered by battery or household current, is durable indoors or outdoors for even the harshest winter weather.

16. **The Simplicity Wheelchair Lift Ramp combines features of a ramp with an electric lift** for economy of space and pocketbook. If you do not have room for a ramp (or it would take up half your yard) and a vertical platform lift is too permanent or two expensive, a Simplicity Wheelchair Lift Ramp may be just right. Roll onto this 8-foot-long ramp, press a button and it raises you to

the height of your door. When it is time to leave, you reverse the process. This durable lift ramp installs indoors or outdoors in about an hour and can be easily uninstalled and taken with you if you move.

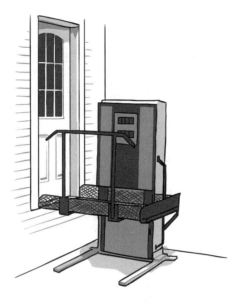

17. **An outdoor stairlift eliminates the need to climb stairs.** If you can walk but need assistance getting up the stairs from driveway to porch, deck, or raised entryway, an outdoor stairlift may be the answer. Just sit on the seat and use hand controls to raise you to the next level.

Before deciding between a ramp or a lift, do your research. Surf the Internet (if you don't have a connection ask family or your local librarian to help you) or contact senior centers, ILCs, or home improvement contractors and building centers that specialize in accessible-housing options for suggestions. To see pictures and demonstration videos of lifts, visit www.Bruno.com.

DOORS, LOCKS, KEYS, AND ENTRY SYSTEMS

18. **Have at least 18 to 24 inches of free space on the side that the door opens.** Be sure that any screen or storm door is hinged on the same side and opens the same way as the main door, or just remove that extra barrier.

19. **Add a bench or package shelf outside exterior doors.** A shelf will also give you a place to set purses, briefcases, and packages so that you do not have to work around them as you try to unlock or open the door. If you have room, a bench inside is also nice; it offers a place to set things or to sit down to remove shoes and boots.

20. **Add a door-closing device.** Once you are through the door, does your wheelchair, walker, or scooter make it difficult to reach the door knob and pull the door closed? You could tie a cord or rope around the door knob and fasten it to a hook mounted at a location that you can reach. Or, if you prefer something a little nicer looking, the E-Z Pull Door Closer™ is an inexpensive solution that is durable, flexible, and almost invisible. Designed by a paraplegic, one end hooks around the door knob, while the other end slips into a holder on the door where it is easy to reach and gives you good leverage for pulling the door closed. You can also remove the puller and take it with you to use on other doors while you are away from home.

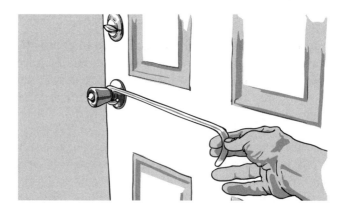

21. **Electric door openers provide maximum independence.** On the expensive side, however, if you are unable to turn keys or open or close doors, opening your door with a remote control or keypad, like you see in public buildings with accessible access, may be the only solution. And when you are inside, you can open the door using a remote control, "buzzing" in your guests, just like you might at an apartment entry. These devices can also be fitted with pressure-sensitive mats or whisper devices for people with severe disabilities.

22. **Replace a standard lock with a keyless entry lock.** Getting in the door is easier if you do not have to fumble with keys. Today there are many alternatives. You can go hi-tech and punch a code into a keypad or use a one-button remote control, similar to the one that opens newer cars. Some can even open the door for you. Ask a locksmith, your security system company, or at a home improvement store about the many options available, or search "keyless locks" on the Internet.

23. **Key turners with built-up handles give you greater leverage** and make turning keys easier. You can make one by placing the head of the key over a comfortable piece of pipe or dowel and securing it with a rubber band wrapped around the key head like a figure-8 or "X," or by using craft putty to fashion a comfortable handle. Ergonomically designed key turners are available in discount catalogs and websites that cater to the elderly such as AidsforArthritis.com.

24. **A lighted key cover makes it easier to find the keyhole** and you can use it to light the sidewalk as you walk. Bright colors and different shapes and textures aid those with visual limitations to identify specific keys.

25. **Install a visual cue for people who are deaf or hard of hearing.** Wire your doorbell to a light on the inside that flashes when the doorbell rings. Any number of commercial beacons and light/ vibration signalers are available from organizations that cater to the deaf and hard of hearing. Ask if you may try out the device before you buy.

26. **Consider a doorbell intercom to make answering the door easier.** If you have difficulty getting to the door to answer it before your visitor leaves, consider replacing your current door bell with an intercom model like you see at security-locked apartments. Place the receiver in a convenient location and when the door bell rings, a buzzer notifies you; you can then talk to the person at the door and let them know you are coming. Add an electric door latch and you can press a button and let the person into your home without getting up. Some models work with your hard-wired telephones, so you can talk to the person at the door from any telephone in the home. You will find these devices at home improvement stores and

from companies that sell home security devices, or your Independent Living Center (ILC) may have options you may try first.

27. **Driveway alerts will signal the arrival of visitors.** Install a wireless driveway alert and when a vehicle enters your driveway, the inside base station will chime, notifying you of visitors and giving you more notice to get to the door. Most devices mount in ground or on a post next to the driveway and send a signal up to 400 feet away. Choose one with an electromagnetic sensor that detects vehicles (mass metal) moving within 3 to 12 feet so that you do not get false alarms from animals moving past the sensor. A sensitivity adjustment is also helpful. You will find these devices at home improvement stores and from companies that sell home security devices.

28. **Use a garage door opener to let guests into the house.** If you have an attached garage and garage door opener, you can use it to let people in when you are lying down or home alone and unable to get to the door.

GARAGE

29. **To accommodate a wheelchair-accessible van in your garage you need a space 15 to 16 feet wide and 7 to 8 feet high**.

30. **Install an automatic garage door opener.** Doing so will give you several advantages:

    - **Easy access to the garage** without having to get out of the vehicle.
    - **An automatic light to welcome you home** and light your way as you exit your vehicle.
    - **A keyless method of entering your home** or as noted above to let others in.

31. **Use high-contrast and reflective tape to mark safe pathways** and keep those areas clear.

32. **Install high-wattage light bulbs** to help you clearly see your way to the door. You may want to consider adding extra light fixtures and motion sensor fixtures.

33. **Clear out unnecessary stuff from your garage.** If you haven't used it in a year, have a garage sale or donate it to charity. For the stuff you need to keep, consider Gladiator® GarageWorks; their heavy-duty plastic tracks are installed along the wall and can be fitted with cabinets, hooks, or baskets that keep items easily visible. This is a nice way to contain the clutter and keep the floor clear and safe. Before purchasing, be sure to use their planning guide to decide which storage options work best for you.

SAFETY

34. **Install automated lighting all around your home to make sure that you can see where you are going.** Motion sensor lights, readily available at hardware and home improvement stores, can be easily installed with a few simple tools. Place them at entryways, in garages, laundry areas, and anywhere you might need light while you have your hands full. If you have a home security system, ask the company that installed it if they have a compatible automatic lighting system that gives you voice or motion sensor lighting all through the house.

35. **A lighted doorbell will help visitors find the bell** and help you find your front door if the overhead light burns out.

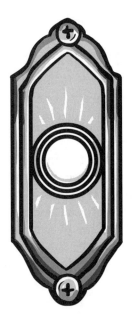

36. **Increase your visibility of visitors outside your door.** Sidelight windows next to the entry door give a clear view of who is outside. If such a window is not practical or you live in a higher crime area, add an additional peep hole 36 to 48 inches from the floor for seated or short adults and children to use. If you have difficulty seeing through a peephole, replace it with a digital Peephole Viewer; its 2.5-inch LCD screen gives you a big, bright image of who is at your door.

37. **Focus light on door locks and house numbers**—the first, so that you can see to get in; the second, so that emergency vehicles can find your house more easily.

38. **Heated floor mats provide traction in winter** so before it snows and your sidewalk is a slippery path, plug a Heat Trak® heated floor mat into your exterior outlet. The mat maintains a 50-degree F temperature that will melt new snow and channel it off to the side for a dry, slip-free walk, for foot traffic only.

39. **Spray a long-acting de-icer on walks before snow and freezing rain occurs.** Effective to 20 degrees F below zero, Bare Ground Deicer™ will keep sidewalks and driveways clear of ice for up to 2 weeks. It is also available in pellets.

40. **Add rubber stair treads to exterior steps.** Not only will they provide better traction but using a contrasting color to the rest of the stairway will help someone with a visual disability differentiate between step and surroundings.

41. **Install solar lights along the entry path to your home** and they will automatically light your way after dark—no switches to remember to turn on. A variety of styles are available that simply push into the ground and operate on the energy from the sun. For raised porches or decks, solar step lights mount on your stair risers, absorb the sun's energy by day and automatically turn on to light your steps for 6 to 8 hours in the evening. Look for these at home improvement centers.

RESOURCES

AARP—Home Fit Guide. This publication contains assessment checklists to help you make your home safer and more accessible as you age.

AARP
601 E Street NW
Washington, DC 20049
Toll free: 888-687-2277
Toll free TTY: 877-434-7598
Toll free Spanish: 877-MAS-DE50 (877-627-3350)
www.AARP.org

Aging in Place video—Exterior Accessibility
Aging in Place Professionals
www.aipathome.com—click on Green Mountain Ranch and select "Exteriors"

PRODUCTS

Ergonomic Key Turners
Aids For Arthritis, Inc.
35 Wakefield Drive
Medford, NJ 08055
Toll free: 800-654-0707
www.AidsforArthritis.com

Aluminum Threshold Ramps
760 S Indiana Avenue
West Bend, WI 53095
Phone: 262-338-3431
Toll free: 888-651-3431
www.discountramps.com

Spray-on De-icer
Bare Ground Systems
2 Sterling Road
Billerica, MA 01862
Toll free: 888-800-8356
www.bareground.com

Products for the Deaf and Hard of Hearing

Center for Communication, Hearing & Deafness
UniversaLink
10243 W. National Avenue
West Allis, WI 53227
Phone: 414-541-5465
Toll free: 800-755-7994
VP toll free: 866-954-9435
TTY: 414-604-7217
www.CCHDWI.org

Digital Peephole Viewer
1998 Ruffin Mill Road
Colonial Heights, VA 23834
Toll free: 800-704-1210
www.firstSTREETonline.com

E-Z Pull Door Closer™
18228 Ackerman Avenue
Port Charlotte, FL 33948
Phone: 941-456-0815
www.E-ZPullDoor.com

Gladiator® Garage Works
Toll free: 866-342-4089
www.gladiatorgarageworks.com

Heat Trak®
85-89 Hazel Street
Paterson, NJ 07503
Phone: 973-357-9797
Toll free: 866-766-9628
www.heattrak.com

Open Sesame Door Systems Inc.
1933 Davis Street, Suite 279
San Leandro, CA 94577
Toll free: 800-673-6911
www.OpenSesameDoor.com

Simplicity Wheelchair Lift Ramp
Raase Lifts, Inc.
W4885 Sunset Lake Court
Sherwood, WI 54169
Toll free: 800-664-8030
www.raaseliftsinc.com

3 in 1 Keyless Entry Lock
16542 Millikan Avenue
Irvine, CA 92606
Toll free: 800-762-7846
www.Smarthome.com

FIVE

All Around the House

When I was diagnosed with MS, I had no idea about the challenges I would face on a daily basis. My home—my sanctuary—seemed to provide a new challenge or frustration every day. Whether it was getting into or out of the shower, unlocking the front door to retrieve the newspaper, or opening up the freezer door to take out something for dinner, I had to stop and think and hope I could do it. The ideas, short cuts, tips, and products I share in this chapter include some of the things I learned through personal experience and trial and error.

Use the information in this chapter to "invent" and discover your own Tips for Making Life Easier™. I hope you'll consider sharing your tip, product, or strategy for Making Life Easier™. What you've "discovered" might help someone else. Email me at Shelley@Making LifeEasier.com.

Accessibility Guidelines

To accommodate a wheelchair, scooter, or walker:

- *Hallways should be 42 to 48 inches wide to keep from scraping knuckles or damaging walls.*
- *A 5-foot circle is required to turn a wheelchair or walker around. A space that is longer than wider (63 × 56 inches) may be even better. (The turning radius of your wheelchair or mobility device should be your guide.)*
- *Doorways should be 32 to 36 inches wide.*
- *Raise electrical outlets to 18 inches from the floor.*
- *Lower light switches, thermostats, and so on to 36 to 44 inches from the floor.*
- *Install grab bars 1.25 to 1.5 inches in diameter, with 1.5 inches from any obstruction such as a wall.*
- *Grab bars and railings should be mounted into studs and support a minimum of 250 pounds.*

To give you some general industry standards and guidelines for accessibility, see the box on page 45. For additional tips and strategies, search the interactive database of tips and products for Making Life Easier™ at www.MakingLifeEasier.com.

DOORS, DOORWAYS, AND DOORKNOBS

42. **Widen doorways**. To give yourself a few extra inches without replacing your door:

43. **Install offset hinges** that swing the door beyond the edge of the doorway exposing the full width of the door opening. You can find these hinges at home improvement stores.

44. **Cut out the door jamb on the bottom half of the door** to add clearance.

45. **Remove doorstops to give yourself an extra three-quarter inch of clearance**. If you absolutely need a doorstop, move it up the wall 3 feet or install the rubber disk style at the level of the door knob, so that it will not be a hazard to mobility devices or people walking by.

46. **If you do not need a solid door in a location, remove the door from its hinges** and you will increase the opening 1 to 1.5 inches. For privacy, use a spring-tension bar (available at bath and hardware stores) to hang a shower curtain over the opening, or you might install folding doors or mount pocket doors on the wall outside the door jamb.

47. **Replace round knobs with lever handles** that can be operated without gripping and turning. If replacing knobs is not an option, wrap a few rubber bands around the knob or purchase easy grip doorknob covers that will give you a better grasp.

48. **Create a lever handle with things you may have around the house:**

    • **Fasten a dowel or piece of small PVC pipe to the doorknob** with a rubber band; be sure to secure both sides of the dowel in a figure-8 pattern.

- **Attach a 4- to 6-inch pipe hanger to the door knob** with a 2-inch-diameter radiator hose clamp. Cover rough edges on the bracket by wrapping it in plastic tape.

49. **Add automatic door openers to heavy doors** or make one by attaching old-fashioned pulleys and weights. It should take no more than 5 pounds of force to open any door.

50. **Disguise doorways and add child-proof latches** to discourage children and those with Alzheimer's, dementia, or other memory issues from entering dangerous areas such as basements and laundry rooms, or exiting exterior doors.

FLOORS AND FLOORING

51. **Hard, smooth surfaces are easier to maneuver than carpet.** Engineered wood floors are attractive and durable; nonslip tile or stone are best in wet areas (kitchen, bathroom, laundry, and entries); natural cork or bamboo offers durability like wood with warmth, cushion, and sound-suppressing qualities similar to carpet.

52. **Carpeted areas should have a dense, low pile that is less than one-half inch.** Conversation areas such as living rooms benefit from the addition of carpeting and curtains that muffle sharp noises and make it easier for someone who is hard of hearing or uses hearing aids to participate in the conversation. Commercial grade carpet and padding provide extra durability under wheels and walkers. Visit a flooring center to see what is available.

53. **Add a contrasting border** to wood, tile, or carpet along the edge of the room.

54. **Inlay a walking path of a different color** to lead the way from room to room.

55. **Change from carpet to a hard surface** when you move from an open living area into a kitchen or hallway.

56. **Contrast flooring with furniture and window coverings** so that someone with limited vision can better see where they are going.

57. **Paint doorways and light switches** in a color in contrast to that of walls.

RAILINGS, STAIRS, AND GRAB BARS

58. **Install railings on both sides of a stairway** so that you have support on either or both sides. Make sure that railings are mounted securely into studs and extend a little beyond the very top step and very bottom step. Railings should be sturdy enough to support 250 pounds at any point.

59. **Paint stair treads a different color than the risers** or install colored treads over carpeted stairs (make sure these are affixed securely) so that you can easily see where each step begins and ends. You might paint every other stair a bright color or mark the edge of steps (or any height change) with contrasting or luminescent paint or tape.

60. **Reduce tripping hazards by closing off any open risers** and reducing any "nosing" (that part of the tread that extends over the riser) to less than 1 inch—either bevel the edge or add a strip of trim or molding to the riser.

61. **Keep stairways well lit**. Increase light bulb wattage and install extra fixtures along the wall if necessary so that all stairs are fully illuminated. You might add tracer lights (like in theaters) to the edge of each stair or mount small low-wattage deck lights (like sidelights at theaters) on or into stair risers to light each step. Check landscaping companies or departments for these inexpensive light fixtures. *Note*: If mounted in the middle of the stair riser, be sure to use a louvered design so that when you are going up the stairs, the lights do not shine in your eyes.

62. **Install stairlifts or elevators to help you get to another floor**. Although expensive, installing a device to get upstairs to a bedroom is less expensive and certainly less traumatic than moving. They are a permanent addition to your house and may affect the resale value of your home. *Before* installing an expensive transport device, see if there is a way to create a bedroom and accessible bathroom on the ground floor that eliminates the need for you to go up or down stairs. The cost

may be similar and will enhance your home's livability as well as value.

63. **Install extra support wherever you need it.** Grab bars have come a long way from the old institutional looking steel bars of even a few years ago. Decorative ergonomic bars that fit the style of your home may be installed almost unobtrusively and sometimes serve dual purposes (towel bar or drapery tie back). Be sure to mount grab bars securely to the studs so that they can support a minimum of 250 pounds.

LIGHTS AND LIGHTING

64. **Replace regular light switches with rocker switches that need little manual** dexterity and work using the back of the hand or elbow.

65. **Purchase a clear plastic light switch extender** if switches are out of reach for children or those who use a wheelchair.

66. **Add sound-, touch-, and motion-activated switches to lights** so that as you enter a room or move through the house the lights turn on and off automatically. Simple fixtures and adapter plugs are available at most hardware or home improvement stores; some even activate security cameras.

67. **Install a whole-house control system** that lets you turn lights on and off throughout the house using a master control, your computer, or a remote, the latter being nice when leaving or returning home in the dark. Ask about trying these at your local Independent Living Center (ILC); once you determine a system that works for you, they can help you order what you need. If you have a home security system, ask the company if they have a compatible automatic lighting system.

LIVING AREAS

68. **Make sure there is 5.5 feet between furniture pieces** to provide easy access for someone using a walker, wheelchair, or scooter; this is also helpful for those with poor vision.

69. **Place furniture in a way so that the backs of heavy pieces can provide support** or give you a place to pause to rest or to adjust to a change in light levels.

70. **Keep low tables and anything with sharp edges out of the path of travel** or cover them with bright towels or tablecloths to help them be seen and to cushion sharp edges.

71. **Place the television on a swivel base or rolling cart** so that it can be moved to see the picture better.

72. **Raise a favorite chair**, if it is too low, to get in or out of easily.

73. **Purchase rubber, plastic, or wooden leg risers** to raise low furniture up a few inches.

74. **Build a box platform for recliners or other chairs (without legs)**. The box platform should be 4 to 5 inches high and have a raised rim (about one-half inch) on the sides and back to keep the chair from slipping or sliding off the platform.

75. **Infrared and looping systems enhance hearing**. Area or whole-room looping systems provide an area of enhanced hearing for those with compatible hearing aids; this is especially helpful in the living or family room where most TV, stereo, and other audio devices are located. Infrared and digital amplifying systems such as TV Ears allow someone who is hard of hearing to adjust the volume of TV and other sound devices so that they can hear without it blasting others out of the room. If you cannot afford a looping system or device, use closed captioning (available on most TV sets) to keep the volume at a reasonable level for others.

76. **Reduce glare to enhance vision.**
    - **Cover shiny desk and table tops.**
    - **Use nonglare floor finishes.**
    - **Reposition mirrors, TVs, and computer monitors.**
    - **Install dimmer switches.**
    - **Use light-filtering curtains on windows so that direct light is reduced without making the room too dark.**

77. **Consider installing battery-operated power shades on key windows** that let you open window coverings with the touch

of a button. You'll find these in decorator shops or window covering sections of home improvement stores.

78. **Change window hardware**:

   - **Add large handles and easy-glide hardware** (with a 5-pound-maximum force) to double-hung windows to make them easier to slide up and down.
   - **Casement windows that crank open are easier to open with one hand**. For better grip, add rubber tips—like those found on the end of canes—to enlarge the ends of the handles or create a custom grip from craft putty.

79. **Use telephones and remote controls with high-contrast, large-print numbers, and buttons**.

   - **Universal remotes with giant buttons are easier for people with poor vision or poor motor control to use**; you will find them online or in electronics stores or departments.
   - **Cordless phones may be moved where you can see more clearly**, whether closer to you or to an area with more light. They also reduce the threat of tripping on wires or cords.
   - **Amplified handsets, captioning, voice-activated, and programmable telephones make phones easier for people with a variety of disabilities to use**.
   - **Contact your local telephone company's special needs department** to ask about phones and services such as free directory assistance and operator-assisted dialing.

You will find more information on using technology to make life easier in Chapter 9, The Accessible Office: Putting Technology to Work for You.

LAUNDRY ROOM

80. **Locate the laundry area on the main floor if possible**. Is there a closet area where a washer and dryer would fit? Think outside the box. Washers and dryers now come in smaller sizes and are stackable. If you choose to stack your machines, make sure you can operate them from a seated position.

81. **Create a comfortable work space**. If you cannot move your laundry area to a more easily accessible main floor location,

create a space with a low shelf for folding clothes, a padded floor mat, and a comfortable chair with reading material where, rather than making multiple trips up and down stairs, you will be comfortable waiting for the wash to be done.

82. **Use a wheeled laundry cart**, hamper, or laundry basket to move heavy clothing (clean or dirty) from room to room. Make your life easier by teaching children to sort and fold their own clothes; use different-colored baskets for sorting darks, lights, and whites.

83. **Install a laundry chute** to a lower-level laundry area. If that is not possible, place a laundry basket or hamper in a location at the bottom of the stairs where your family can just toss dirty clothes; in this way, you do not need to carry heavy baskets of clothing down to the laundry area. Once cleaned, let family members retrieve and put away their own clothing.

84. **Replace a top-loading washer with a front-loading model**. A front-loading machine is easier to use by someone in a wheelchair and has the added benefit of using less water. Keep in mind that you cannot add forgotten dirty items to a front-loading washing machine once it has been started.

85. **Raise your washer and dryer**. Build a platform under your front-loading washer and dryer to raise them 18 inches off the floor; this height is more comfortable for both people who are standing and for those in a seated position. Build a drawer into your platform to store laundry or other supplies. Be sure to add child locks on cabinets and drawers that hold potentially harmful products.

86. **Vent the dryer to outside**—especially if it is a gas dryer. And, don't forget to clean out dryer vents to the outside once or twice a year.

87. **Be kind to yourself and the environment**—use less toxic and fragrance-free products. Many natural products are highly concentrated, so a little goes a long way. "Green living" books give directions for making nontoxic laundry products using vinegar, baking soda, and other things you have around the

house. You'll save money too. Here are a few suggestions to get you started:

- **Nontoxic laundry detergent:**
  - 1 cup soap flakes
  - 1/2 cup washing soda (1 cup if you have hard water)
  - 1/2 cup Borax
- **Add one-half cup white distilled vinegar to rinse as a fabric softener.**
- **Instead of using chlorine bleach**, presoak dingy white clothes in a washer filled with enough water to cover clothes and one-half cup of hydrogen peroxide; or add one-half cup of lemon juice to wash cycle.

CLOSETS, CONTAINERS, AND STORAGE

88. **Lower some closet bars or install closet organizers** that adjust to provide multiple hanging levels (higher and lower) and bring clothing within reach of someone who is seated. Power- and lift-assist closet bars that lower upper closet bars to you then raise them out of the way are now available. Be sure to test these devices fully loaded with clothing before purchasing.

89. **Install adjustable shelving to fit your space and needs**. Closet systems by California Closets®, Rubbermaid®, Elfa®, or other companies, let you pick and choose elements such as shelves and slide out drawers and baskets to design a space that will fit your exact needs. Find closet systems at your local discount, department, or container store or online retailers.

90. **Use clear storage bins so that you can see what is inside**. Clear plastic drawers or wire baskets provide easy to see and access storage throughout the house. Add large-print labels to exposed ends to help you (or someone assisting you) know what goes inside.

91. **Store things close to where you need them**, and in logical places. Keep all the gardening equipment together; store the bike helmets next to the bikes; create an equipment storage area with cubbies and hooks to hold sports gear (if inside, you might even want to add an exhaust fan and a dehumidifier to

reduce or eliminate odors.) Put the heaviest and most used items on the shelves that are easiest to reach.

92. **Store some things outside**. Consider a deck box for children's toys or a storage shed for gardening tools. Consult your local home improvement store for options.

ENVIRONMENTAL CONSIDERATIONS

93. **Install a programmable thermostat** so that you can set the temperature for different days or parts of days. Be sure to choose a thermostat with an easy-to-read display window, large programming buttons, and install it lower on the wall (36 to 44 inches from the floor) so that someone in a seated position may see the display and operate it. Some thermostats even come with a remote control so that you can control the temperature from a short distance away.

94. **Replace your current thermostat with a large-print model** that has easy-to-read numbers. Raised numbers and a dial that clicks at every 2-degree setting helps those who are blind or with severe vision challenges. *Note*: Thermostats require professional installation.

95. **Change your furnace filter every 3 months** to keep your indoor air cleaner and your furnace operating more efficiently. Use a filter with a high MERV rating to reduce the amount of dirt and dust circulating through the air vents.

96. **Vacuum frequently.** To keep dust mites and other respiratory hazards out from underfoot and in the air you breathe, vacuum carpets and floors once or twice a week with a good-quality sealed, True-HEPA, or "zero emissions" vacuum cleaner.

97. **If building or remodeling a home, consider installing a central vacuum system.** Although expensive, central vacuum systems have been clinically proven by the University of California at Davis to reduce allergy symptoms by as much as 61%. Because of their larger, more powerful suction, they are not only more effective at removing dirt, dust mites, pollen, dander, and other allergens than conventional vacuums, but they completely

remove them from living areas to a canister usually located in the garage. Ask a building or remodeling contractor for more information.

98. **Clean the air with a HEPA air cleaner**. HEPA air filters remove 99.97% of particles from the air, making your home environment safer for those with asthma, respiratory illnesses, allergies, and chemical sensitivities. Avoid air cleaners that emit ozone, a known lung irritant.

99. **Leave shoes at the door** to avoid tracking in dirt, molds and, more importantly, herbicide and pesticide residues.

100. **Steam clean carpets and furniture regularly.** Skip the chemicals, the steam is enough to kill germs and bacteria; the suction will pull out the dirt.

101. **Use zero-VOC (volatile organic compound) paints and varnishes** and nontoxic products for everything from cleaning products to air fresheners, candles, and even flea and tick treatments for your pets. Use organic fertilizers and herbicides.

102. **Let dry-cleaning air outside** or in the garage for at least 24 hours, and let any new fabrics, drapes, upholstered furniture, or carpet off-gas for at least 2 to 3 weeks before bringing them into the house. *Note*: Carpet must be rolled out flat to off-gas.

103. **Ventilate.** Run exhaust fans in the kitchen and bathroom, and vent all appliances to the outside.

Studies show that indoor air pollution can far exceed outdoor pollution. For more tips for making your home cleaner and healthier, see "8 Tips for a Healthier Home" at www.MakingLife Easier.com.

104. **Filter your water.** Install a good-quality water filter on your kitchen faucet or sink, or use a filtering pitcher (like a Britta®), for drinking water.

105. **Since an abundance of chemicals can enter your body through your skin, be sure to filter your shower water as well**. If you have more than one or two faucets you want

to filter, ask your plumbing contractor about whole-house water filters; it costs more initially but pays for itself in the long run.

GENERAL SAFETY

106. **Make your home familiar and safe.** Avoid the urge to rearrange the furniture—keeping everything in the same place is an important strategy for people who are blind, with poor vision, mobility impairments, and memory issues. For safety purposes, install locks on doors and cabinets containing medicines, toxic substances, and dangerous utensils or tools; remove electrical appliances from your bathroom; install non-scald faucets, or set your water heater temperature to 120 °C (do not do both or water will not be hot enough to kill bacteria when you wash); install grab bars and automatic lighting—in this way you will help prevent accidents around the home.

107. **Schedule time regularly for home safety and maintenance checks** and you will never be left in a crisis situation.

    • **Change batteries** in smoke detectors, smoke alarms, and your thermostat once a year
    • **Change exterior light bulbs every fall,** before the bad weather arrives
    • **Vacuum the coils on the back of your refrigerator** at least twice a year; this will help it be more efficient too
    • **To reduce the risk of fire, clean out the dryer vent hose** (that is vented to the outside) at least twice a year

108. **Install a whole-house intercom or use baby monitors.** If you have a baby in the house or a loved one is prone to wandering or confined to bed, save running back and forth checking on them by installing a multistation intercom or monitor. Place a monitor in each room, plug it into the electric outlet, and with the touch of a button, you can communicate with any or all of the others. (Range is usually about 1,500 feet which covers the average house.) These systems are available at home improvement stores. If you have a home security system, the company might offer an add-on. To try an intercom system before you

buy, contact your local ILC to see if they have one in their loan closet.

109. **Install an alert system.** Smoke and carbon monoxide detectors, weather monitors, telephones, doorbells, burglar alarms, and baby monitors, all can be attached to a transmitter that flashes and gets your attention even if you cannot hear the alarm. Some even work with a vibrating receiver you wear as a watch band. If you have a security system, ask about wiring in visual (flashing lights) as well as audible alerts.

110. **Invest in remote home control and management systems.** These systems are expensive but if you are severely disabled, or even if you are not, it is nice to be able to make and receive phone calls, unlock doors, turn on lights, and control the temp- erature, TV, and audio devices remotely without having to get up or ask for assistance. There are numerous products and remote control systems on the market that allow you to auto- mate or manually control many of the daily functions of your home. For example: Plug a lamp into a simple receiver plugged into a wall outlet, and turn the light on from a master receiver or from anywhere in the home via remote control; open a garage door and exterior and interior home lights go on automatically; opening a door lock triggers the security system to deactivate, the lights to turn on, and send a notification to a PC or cell phone via the Internet to let you know the kids are home; or a motion detector can trigger an outdoor security light and a webcam that would allow the home dweller to monitor the home from a bedroom or while away.

Here are just a few systems to consider. All offer the benefits of starting small—with the front door, lights, or garage—and adding on to the system over time.

- **X10**—This technology has been around for several decades now. It uses existing wiring in your home to transmit signals from the master control transmitter to receivers attached to lamps and other electrical devices throughout your home. You may program up to 256 channels or distinct devices to go on or off, dim or brighten, and so on. Multiple devices may be programmed to operate together such as opening a door latch and turning on a light. Regardless of the manufacturer, all X10 compatible products can be freely mixed and matched, and so you can add on to your system as needs dictate.

- **Z-Wave**—This is a wireless technology built into a number of electronic devices. By adding or "pairing" this technology with home electronics such as lighting, climate control, and security systems, it is possible to automate or manually control and monitor a single device or group of devices, in a single room or throughout the entire home. One of the benefits of Z-Wave is that it works wirelessly and has the ability to function in older houses lacking a neutral wire. Z-Wave devices can also be monitored and controlled from outside of the home by way of a gateway that combines Z-Wave with broadband Internet access.

- **INSTEON** combines wireless radio frequency with your home's existing electrical wiring to transmit signals to various devices. Using dual-signal transmission reduces possible interference and strengthens the signal. INSTEON has a two-way repeater system, and is compatible with X10 products.

Only you can determine which system and options are best for you. So, read about the advantages and disadvantages of the different systems and, if possible, talk with various users. Also, know that as technology improves more options and better systems will become available. If you feel you would benefit from this technology, ask your rehabilitation therapist or ILC for more information about the products and possible funding sources. Also see if you can try the system you are interested in before you purchase it.

111. Keep reachers wherever they come in handy. Many different types of reachers are available to relieve the strain of bending, stretching, or stooping. Some models have pistol grips, others work like a giant pair of tongs, and some fold compactly to take with you. I don't know what I would do without my reachers—from my wheelchair I can reach dishes and glasses, put groceries away, hang up clothes in the closet, get things out of the refrigerator, and pick up almost anything that has fallen to the floor. I have different reachers for different purposes. One of my favorites is the TeleStik which comes with a magnetic, a sticky, and a hook end. It is lightweight and slim enough to get into tight spaces. For a description of different reachers and their uses see *8 Ways to Get a Grip with Reachers* at www. MakingLifeEasier.com.

112. **Carry a portable magnifier with you.** In addition to an old-fashioned, inexpensive magnifying glass, numerous hand-held devices are on the market today to help people who struggle to read standard print. These portable devices slip easily into a pocket or clip onto your belt loop ready to enlarge reading material, package inserts, recipes, and so on. Portable readers like the Intel® Reader scan text and read text aloud. There is even "an app for that;" ZoomReader, which turns your Smartphone into a portable magnifier at a very low price. Ask your eye doctor, occupational or rehab therapist, or ILC about the Amigo, Pebble, or other portable magnifying and reading devices.

RESOURCES

AARP offers a number of free publications for making life easier as one ages and faces limitations. You will find helpful checklists for making your home more accessible with various limitations in their

Home Improvement section; see "How Well is Your Home Caring for You?"
AARP
601 E Street, NW
Washington DC, 20049
Toll free: 888-OUR-AARP (888-687-2277)
Toll free TTY: 877-434-7598
Toll free Spanish: 877-MAS-DE50 (877-627-3350)
www.AARP.org

The American Lung Association provides information on how to breathe easier in your home.
Health House®
3000 Kelly Lane
Springfield, IL 62711
Phone: 217-787-5864
Toll free: 800-788-5864
www.HealthHouse.org

Healthy Home Institute® is a comprehensive informational resource for maintaining a healthy home environment.
The Healthy House Institute®, LLC
13998 West Hartford Drive
Boise, ID 83713
www.HealthyHomeInstitute.com

PRODUCTS

Alert Systems
Center for Communication, Hearing, and
Deafness—UniversaLink
10243 W National Avenue
West Allis, WI 53227
Phone: 414-541-5465
Toll free: 800-755-7994
VP toll free: 866-954-9435
TTY: 414-604-7217
www.CCHDWI.org

AllergyBuyersClub.com / SleepBuyersClub.com
Boston Green Goods, Inc.
45 Braintree Hill Park, Suite 300
Braintree, MA 02184
Phone: 781-419-5500
Toll free: 888-236-7231
www.allergybuyersclub.com

Amigo or Pebble Magnifier
Enhanced Vision
5882 Machine Drive
Huntington Beach, CA 92649
Toll free: 888-811-3161
www.enhancedvision.com

Decorative, Ergonomic Grab Bars
Great Grabz™
4535 Domestic Ave, Suite D
Naples, FL 34104
Phone: 239-403-4722
Toll free: 866-478-4722
www.GreatGrabz.com

Furniture Leg Risers
Walter Drake®
250 City Center
Oshkosh, WI 54906
Toll free: 800-525-9291
www.wdrake.com

HEPA Air Cleaner, Vacuums, Water Filters, and more
AllergyBuyersClub.com/SleepBuyersClub.com
Boston Green Goods, Inc.
45 Braintree Hill Park, Suite 300
Braintree, MA 02184
Phone: 781-419-5500
Toll free: 888-236-7231
www.allergybuyersclub.com

HEPA Vacuums
Miele, Inc.
9 Independence Way
Princeton, NJ 08540
Toll free: 800-640-2623
www.Miele.com

Home Marketplace
PO Box 3670
Oshkosh, WI 54903
Toll free: 800-356-3876
TTY: 920-231-5506
www.TheHomeMarketplace.com

INSTEON
Smarthome
16542 Millikan Avenue
Irvine, CA 92606
Toll free: 800-762-7846
www.smarthome.com

Intel© Reader
HumanWare
PO Box 800
Champlain, NY 12919
Toll free: 800-722-3393
www.humanware.com

Light Switch Extender
Dynamic Living
95 West Dudley Town Road
Bloomfield, CT 06002
Toll free: 888-940-0605
www.Dynamic-Living.com

Power Lift Closet Bars
Home improvement stores or
Dynamic Living—AdaptMy.com
95 West Dudley Town Road
Bloomfield, CT 06002
Toll free: 866-993-0783
www.AdaptMy.com

Residential Elevators
Waupaca Elevator Company, Inc.
1726 N Ballard Road
Appleton, WI 54911
Toll free: 800-238-8739
www.WaupacaElevator.com

Sound Enhancing Looping Systems
Center for Communication, Hearing, and
Deafness—UniversaLink
10243 W National Avenue
West Allis, WI 53227
Phone: 414-541-5465
Toll free: 800-755-7994
VP toll free: 866-954-9435
TTY: 414-604-7217
www.CCHDWI.org

Stair Lift Videos
www.Bruno.com

TeleStik™
Cougar Mountain Marketing Corporation
15355—24th Avenue, Suite 800-575
Surrey, BC, Canada V4A 2H9
Phone: 604-542-2982
www.telestik.com

Wireless TV Listening Systems
As seen on TV, in mail-order catalogs or from
LS & S (Learning, Sight, and Sound)
145 River Rock Drive
Buffalo, NY 14207
Toll free: 800-468-4789
Toll free TTY: 866-317-8533
www.LSSproducts.com

X10
Smarthome
16542 Millikan Avenue
Irvine, CA 92606
Toll free: 800-762-7846
www.smarthome.com

ZoomReader iTunes app
ai squared
PO Box 669
Manchester Center, VT 05255
Phone: 802-362-3612
Toll free: 800-859-0270
www.aisquared.com

Z-Wave
1778 McCarthy Boulevard
Milpitas, CA 95035
Phone: 408-262-9003
www.z-wave.com

SIX

The Accessible Kitchen

The kitchen is usually the heartbeat of the home. Even today, with our children grown with families of their own, whenever the "kids" are home, the kitchen is where everyone congregates. Generally, the most expensive room in the house to remodel is the kitchen, so as I lost my physical abilities, I tried to modify the way I did things. My husband and I organized the kitchen to make it easier for me to participate. I sat on a stool when I was cooking at the stove. I put the silverware in a tray that we kept near the table to eliminate the need to carry the silverware to the table.

As it became more difficult for me to participate in meal preparation, cooking, and cleanup, I tried to stay involved and do what I could. I didn't want to abdicate my responsibility just because of my limitations. So, my husband and I taught the

Accessibility Guidelines

To accommodate a wheelchair, scooter, or walker:

- *Kitchen aisles should be 46 to 48 inches wide.*
- *You will need a 5-foot turning circle at both ends; a space that is longer than wider (63 × 56 inches) may be even better. (The turning radius of your wheelchair or mobility device should be your guide.)*
- *Doorways should be a 32 to 36 inches wide. Remove narrower doors wherever possible and replace pantry doors with curtains, folding doors, or pocket doors.*
- *Keep things within reach of a seated person:*
  24 inches or less to the front or side
  No more than 12 inches from the floor or 52 inches high.
- *Raise the cabinet toe space to 9 inches.*

kids how to use small appliances and knives safely. After dinner, I supervised the kids while they washed the dishes and swept the floor, using techniques and devices that made it easier for them to manage.

I hope the ideas and suggestions in this chapter help and guide you as you adapt your kitchen to your needs. If you have any questions or would like more ideas for managing mealtime, visit www.Making LifeEasier.com and search our database of tips.

OPEN FLOOR PLAN

The most important thing about having an accessible kitchen is having enough room to move around without hindrance. Aisles should be wide enough for two people to pass each other or for a wheelchair to turn around. Appliances, countertops, sinks, and faucets should be within easy reach for someone in a seated position. Cabinets and drawers should open easily. Check out the products described in this chapter at home improvement or kitchen design stores to see what's available to make your life easier. See the Accessibility Guidelines on p. 65 for dimensions to keep in mind for the kitchen.

FLOORING CHOICES

113. **Use nonskid flooring and finishes**. Wood or nonskid stone or tile floors stand up better in heavy-duty work spaces like the kitchen and are much more sanitary than carpet.

114. **Try cork flooring** if you want the cushion and warmth of carpet along with sound-dampening qualities. Cork is also anti-static, fire resistant, *and* good for the environment since harvesting cork does not kill the tree.

115. **Apply nonslip coatings to existing floors**. If you cannot afford to replace the floor, there are products on the market that can be applied to existing tile or stone flooring that will prevent slipping yet will not damage the surface or wear off easily. Ask about these at any good flooring store.

116. **Add a contrasting border** to delineate where the floor ends and the wall begins.

117. **Provide visual cues to work spaces** by changing the color of the wood or tile in front of the sink and stove; as part of the overall design of the floor, this can be a nice decorative touch.

118. **A quick and inexpensive way to provide contrast between surfaces is to apply painter's tape** (the blue tape you find in paint stores) to the wall where it meets the floor. Painter's tape is designed to come off without damaging paint or woodwork, and you can outline doors and cabinet edges with it as well.

119. **Avoid busy patterns in flooring.** Solid-colored linoleum or tile is less visually confusing than patterned or checkerboard styles. Some experts recommend laying tile at an angle. They feel that a diamond pattern points the way, creating more of a visual walkway than multiple straight rows of tile. Adjacent carpeted areas should be plain or a simple multicolor (tweed), with a dense weave and low pile (less than one-half inch).

120. **When installing a carpet next to a bare wood or tiled floor, inset the carpet** so that there will be no lip or other tripping hazard between hard and carpeted surfaces.

APPLIANCES, TOOLS, AND EQUIPMENT

This section lists just a few things you might want to consider to make your kitchen more accessible. Many appliances, by many manufacturers, are now being designed with all users—standing, sitting, one-handed or two-handed, able or frail—in mind. Visit a home improvement store or kitchen design center to see what's new. Choose a store that has a demonstration kitchen where you can try out different styles and determine which features work best for you.

121. **When you purchase new appliances, keep accessibility features in mind:**

    • **Instead of a traditional stove/oven combination, install a stovetop** 30 to 32 inches high, with front-mounted, child-safe controls, over an open cabinet that allows a minimum of 24 inches of knee space (high and wide) for the cook in a wheelchair. Wall racks under the stovetop will provide handy storage for the most-often-used utensils.

- **A wall oven mounted 18 inches off the floor or at countertop height is easier to use**—no matter what your height. Add a pull-out shelf underneath to slide hot dishes onto.

- **Purchase side-hinged appliances.** Not only does a side-hinged oven take up less space in the kitchen but it is safer since there is no bending and reaching over a hot oven door. Some appliances come with doors that slide to the side.

- **Use a side-by-side refrigerator.** Having both the freezer and the refrigerator section accessible from top to bottom is easier for everyone, even children, to access. Place the most frequently used items within easy reach in the shallow shelves on the door or in slide-out baskets and drawers.

- **Consider purchasing a drawer-style dishwasher.** Maytag® makes one with two drawers; use the clean dishes from one drawer while you put dirty dishes in the other. Or, reduce the need to bend over to load or unload your dishwasher by mounting your dishwasher higher, with the base 12 to 18 inches off the floor. Create an extra storage space underneath the dishwasher by installing a drawer that can hold detergent or rarely used items.

- **Look for "talking" appliances.** Many appliances now speak nearly every operation and setting, such as "rinse" or "dry." Ask about appliances with these features at a kitchen design center.

- **When purchasing a new microwave oven,** consider getting a convection model that will bake foods like a traditional oven but in a fraction of the time, with less energy and heat.

- **Consider a trash compactor** to make taking the trash out easier, or use wheeled trash cans that roll out to be emptied.

122. **Place frequently used appliances on countertops.** Microwave ovens, toasters, or blenders are much easier to use if they are at countertop height instead of over the stove or inside a cabinet. Cover the appliances with decorative covers if you don't like them sitting out or create an appliance "garage" with a retractable tambour door to hide them; kits are available online.

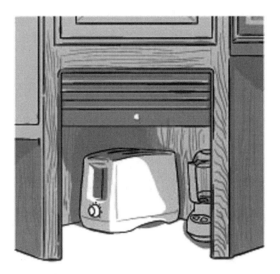

123. **Use electrical appliances rather than manual ones whenever possible**, including food processors, standing mixers, blenders, and under-the-cabinet can and jar openers.

124. **Use a toaster oven for most baking and broiling.** In addition to the countertop oven being easier to reach and use, you will not be heating up the whole kitchen to bake a small meal. Find smaller baking pans and casserole dishes that fit these smaller ovens in mail order catalogs like Walter Drake®.

125. **Slow cookers** now allow you to cook *and* store food in the same container making cooking and cleanup easier.

126. **Electric "cocoa-latte" hot drink makers** that heat milk, water, soups, and other liquids and dispense them with a nozzle are fast, easy, safe to use, and keeps cleanup to a minimum.

127. **Consider suspending a mirror over the stove** (like they use in cooking demonstrations) so that someone in a seated position can see what's happening to the food on the cook top. Look for lightweight, unbreakable mirrors in toy or auto departments.

128. **Add additional task lighting where you need it.** Install strip lighting under counters, spot lighting on ceilings, and put higher-wattage bulbs in stove hoods. If that is not enough light, consider adding a goose-neck, clamp-on light to the

edge of a cabinet to throw extra light on your work space so that you can see what you are doing more easily.

129. **Install controls under the counter**. Install on/off switches for lights, fans, and even the garbage disposal under the counter where they are handy for all to reach. It is convenient to have an electrical outlet at this level also. *Note*: If you have small children, or they visit, be sure to use appropriate childproofing measures.

130. **Create colored or raised markings on control knobs**. Use colored tapes, puffy paint, glue, or stick-on "bumps" to create raised markings for standard settings on appliances, faucets, and other frequently used items. A combination of color coding and raised tactile markings works best. Knobs that click will give auditory cues to their settings—one click is high, two is medium, and so on.

131. **To operate an electric can opener with one hand**, place the can on a piece of Styrofoam^{TM} that is the correct height for the can to connect with the cutting blades. Use the Styrofoam to hold the can while you operate the can opener. There are also other types of automatic can and jar openers. Contact your local Independent Living Center (ILC) to see what kinds of automatic can and jar openers are available for you to try.

132. **Create a mixing bowl holder** by cutting a circle out of a heavy wood block the diameter of your bowl, or stabilize the bowl by placing it on a washcloth or rubber shelf liner inside a drawer.

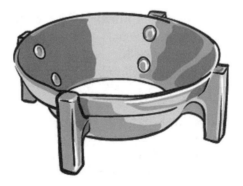

133. **Use decorative pots and pans that double as serving pieces**. Display the ones you use most often on top of the stove instead of putting them back into the cupboard where you have to reach for and lift them.

134. **Store tools where you are most likely to use them**. Hang pots and pans near the stove, arrange cooking utensils in a decorative crock on the counter, install door racks and hooks for towels, pot holders and other frequently used items, and store dishes near the sink or dishwasher.

135. **Purchase "suction ware" to make food preparation and eating easier**. Whether you are one-handed, have tremors, or have a weak grip, suction-bottomed cutting boards, mixing bowls, kitchen tools, and dinnerware will keep everything right where you want it. A low-cost alternative is to use a piece of rubber or waffle-like shelf liner under bowls and dishes to keep them from slipping. Some newer mixing bowls and tools now come with nonslip bottoms; see the latest at your nearest kitchen store.

136. **Replace old kitchen tools with newer ergonomic models**. Everything from mixing spoons to peelers and graters now come with large, easy-to-grip, comfort handles. Check out your choices at OXO.com. Rocker knives with curved rather than straight blades, such as the ULU, work with cutting bowls that keep food contained or as an easier way for someone with limitations to cut food at the table. Check out your nearest kitchen store or in catalogs for seniors or Websites such as aidsforarthritis.com or firstSTREETonline.com.

137. **Replace a standard cutting board with one that better meets your needs.**

    - **If you are one-handed** or otherwise have difficulty holding an item in place, choose a cutting board with metal tines on the surface to hold what you are cutting. You can make your own by driving two 3- to 4-inch galvanized nails through your existing cutting board and adding slats of wood on one corner to keep food from slipping off. The nails should be placed a couple of inches in from the edge and be countersunk (when the nail is driven all the way into the wood, use a tool to drive the nail head in a little further so it does not stick out or rub on your counter).

- **If you have difficulty seeing what you are cutting,** purchase brightly colored cutting boards designed to reduce cross-contamination of meat with raw fruits and vegetables. Cut dark- or bright-colored items on a light board and light items on a dark board.
- **Specialty and mail-order catalogs now offer any number of special utensils** that allow you to hold an onion, tomato, or other small item and cut it evenly. In addition to holding items in place, they provide a guide for your knife, and protect your fingers.

138. **Use a wheeled utility cart** to transport food, dishes, and heavy items around the kitchen and to the dining area. A cart will also provide a little extra support and stability as you walk.

COUNTERS AND CABINETS

139. **If you are building or remodeling, create a tight work triangle.** Place the stove, sink, and refrigerator within close proximity but with counter space in between for placing things to be trans-ferred from one area to another. This eliminates unnecessary moving around, especially with hot food or heavy dishes.

140. **Install cabinets at various heights for different tasks.** Have at least one work station 27 inches off the floor that is open underneath and accessible to someone in a seated position. A desk that is used for one person becomes a "just right" work space for another. If you cannot physically change the counter height, consider getting a stool (on wheels) that allows someone to sit while working.

141. **Widen aisles by replacing some of the lower cabinets with bathroom cabinets,** which are only 18 inches deep instead of the usual 24 inches. Do this on one side of the kitchen and you have gained 6 inches. Since bathroom cabinets are also shorter, you may choose to use these as your accessible work station, or raise them up with a higher 9-inch toe space (the space between the bottom of the cabinet and the floor) under-neath. Determine what works best for you.

142. **Install full-extension drawers and shelves in base cabinets**. Slide-out drawers and shelves in lower cabinet areas are more useable for everyone and eliminate the need to get down on your knees and crawl inside. If you are not in the market for new cabinets with these features already installed, home improvement stores sell wire inserts. For something sturdier, consider custom wood and laminate sliding drawers for your existing cabinets.

143. **Bring some cabinets down to the countertop height**. This provides an easily accessible place for children to reach their cereal and breakfast bowls. It also creates a convenient location for people who are seated or have poor grip to slide items out onto the countertop to prepare a meal.

144. **Consider adding motorized cabinets**. The cabinet unit is mounted on a support and at the touch of a button it can be raised or lowered for access by people of different heights. Though expensive, these make it possible for someone in a wheelchair to have full access to cabinets and supplies while cooking, yet the cabinets can be raised to an ordinary height when someone else is working in the kitchen.

145. **Weighted shelving inserts** fit inside your cabinets. These are counterbalanced so that they pull down or lift up with very little effort and provide easy access to cabinet contents.

146. **Add a roll-out/pull-out cabinet if you have a narrow empty space next to the refrigerator**. As with a side-by-side refrigerator canned goods and foodstuffs, and even food prep and storage containers can be located at eye level for various family members. Another option is to add an inexpensive, over-the-door wire shelving unit to hold cans and boxes.

147. **Replace any round pull knobs** with "C" or "D" shaped handles (shaped like the letter suggests)—available at your local hardware or home improvement store—that can be opened with little effort for people with weak or painful hands. To make an existing knob into a lever handle, secure a cane or furniture leg tip over the knob, drill a hole the size of a wooden dowel and push the dowel through the hole to create a lever.

148. **Install easy-glide and self-closing hardware on all cabinet drawers and doors**. Many people have trouble grasping and pulling open doors and drawers. Your local hardware or home improvement store has all you need to make your doors close softly and your drawers glide open and close more easily.

149. **Install slide-away cabinet doors**. They now make hardware for cabinet doors that allows the door, when fully opened, to then be slid back into the cabinet, parallel to the side walls. This allows easy access to the cabinet without having to constantly open and close the doors.

150. **Use contrasting color cabinet doors and countertops**. Dark counters and doors over lighter cabinets and floors help older people or those with low vision see where the counter or cabinet ends and the floor begins.

FAUCETS AND SINKS

151. **Remove the cabinet under the sink** to allow someone in a wheelchair to reach it easier. Be sure to cover hot-water pipes to avoid knee burns; this can be done with an angled piece of plywood, a cloth drape, foam pipe insulation, or a fanciful plastic coil wrapped around the plumbing pipe. If you prefer the look of a cabinet but need the open space underneath, carefully deconstruct the doors and supports, and remove the cabinet floor. Then reattach the center post and kickplates to the doors. When closed, the cabinet will have a similar appearance to all the others.

152. **Locate the kitchen sink at a 45-degree angle in the corner of the kitchen counter**, ideally with clear floor space below, low enough (30 to 32 inches from the floor) so that the sink and faucet are within easy reach of someone who is seated.

153. **Mount the kitchen faucet at the side to make it easier to reach for someone in a seated position, and for children.**

154. **Choose single-lever faucet handles that can be operated with one hand**. Choose a model that you can operate with a closed fist. Or, install no-touch motion sensor faucets that turn on

and off automatically when you place your hands under the faucet. (These faucets are nice for those who have trouble gripping and turning but also for those who tend to forget to turn the water off.) Inexpensive, no-touch adapters that fit most existing faucets are readily available at home improvement stores or online.

155. **Install faucets with pull-out, hand-held spray nozzles** that allow you to direct the water where you want it.

156. **Add a pot-filler faucet near the stove** that folds out of the way when not in use. Having a water source at the stove is handy when you need to add a little liquid while cooking and will reduce the need for transporting heavy pots of water from the sink. An alternative is to use a spaghetti cooker or other pot with a built-in strainer to carry and cook your food in; let someone else fill and empty the pot of water for you.

DINING AREAS

157. **Use color contrast to help you see what you are eating.** Choose dishes and flatware that contrast with the table or table linens, placing light-colored dishes on dark tables or tablecloths and dark or brightly colored dishes on light-colored tables or linens. You might even want to have two sets of dishes, one to serve light-colored foods, another to serve darker-colored meals.

158. **Bright-colored placemats and flatware increase visibility at the table.** Choose flatware with larger, easy-to-grip handles in a color that contrasts with the linens.

159. **Divided plates make eating easier.** So if someone has difficulty seeing or has tremors, and getting food onto the fork or spoon is difficult, consider using divided plates with a nonslip bottom. Make almost any surface nonslip with rubber shelf liner available in almost any kitchen section of any home improvement store.

160. **Add a Lazy Susan to the table.** Keep salt, pepper, napkins, and other regularly used items handy by placing them on a Lazy Susan; a simple spin brings everything within reach of everyone at the table.

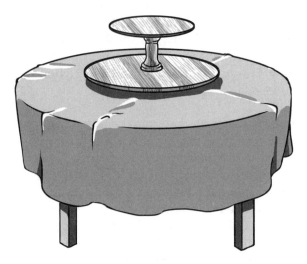

161. **Protect upholstered dining room chairs from spills**. Keep food and beverage spills from ruining your good dining room chairs by covering them with heavy-duty clear plastic covers. Purchase these ready-made or buy plastic by the roll at fabric or hardware stores.

162. **Use an extra-deep lap tray** if one is unable to sit at the table. When someone has a tremor, difficulty holding or controlling utensils, or is in a wheelchair or bed, an extra inch of tray height will keep food and dishes from sliding off onto a lap or the floor.

LIGHTING

163. **Make sure you have enough light**. Someone who is 80 years old needs at least three times the light to see than a 20-year-old. Use bright bulbs in overhead lights to avoid shadows that might cause tripping hazards. If more light is needed, install additional task lighting or try a goose-necked fixture, perhaps with a magnifying mirror (like the ones architects use), over the main food preparation area.

164. **Install LED task lighting under all upper cabinets** where it will light the work space without shinning in your eyes. Consider a row of tube or "chaser lights" around the edge of any peninsulas or islands so that they can be easily seen in low light.

165. **Increase natural light**. In addition to illuminating the space, natural light has profound psychological benefits for everyone. Enlarge windows or add French doors and skylights to bring sunlight into the room. Also, sheer curtains will muffle sharp outdoor sounds without reducing the light too much.

ORGANIZING

166. **Place frequently used or heavy items in lower cabinets**. Consider adding pull-out boards under the countertop as a step between shelves and counter, slide-out shelves in the cabinets for easier access to items, or spring-assisted shelving to help raise heavy items to countertop height. See these options demonstrated at a quality kitchen or cabinet shop.

167. **Store dishes vertically** within easy reach. Instead of stacking heavy dishes, stand them on end. (Do the same with baking sheets and pans.) You can purchase cabinets with this feature or create your own by adding small dowels to create a space to stand plates in existing cabinets. Inexpensive, ready-made inserts may be found at discount stores or mail-order catalogs. To make access to dishes even easier, move them to a lower cabinet that is easier to reach and consider removing doors to this heavily used area.

168. **Install cabinet, drawer, and pull-down, under-the-cabinet organizers**. It is much easier (and safer in the case of knives) to find things if you have a place for everything and everything in its place. Standard organizers are made for drawers, cabinets, pantries, and more. See what is available at a kitchen design store online or in your home town; mail order catalogs often offer inexpensive versions. To make your own low-cost drawer organizers, use binder clips and an assortment of flat boxes and containers and clip them together.

169. **Use lightweight baskets inside cupboards** to keep small things tidy and within reach.

170. **Use a Lazy Susan or turntable in the refrigerator and in cupboards** to bring items to you rather than having to reach for them.

SAFETY

171. **Consider putting child safety locks on all cupboards and cabinets.** In addition to keeping children out of hazardous materials, these are helpful for keeping people with Alzheimer's disease and dementia safe as well.

172. **Get in the habit of closing cabinet doors and drawers** when you are not actively using them; this will cut down the risk of someone else walking into them. Mark the end and inside edges of doors and drawers with strips of bright-colored tape so that someone with poor vision can easily discern that the door or drawer is open. Safety yellow/orange or red is often a good choice but use the color most visible to the one with the visual impairment.

173. **Use lights and vibrating alarms to remind you that you are cooking.**

   • **Turn the oven light or the light over your stove on** to remind you that you have something in the oven.
   • **Attach a Sonic Boom Alarm Clock with Bed Shaker to a lamp in the kitchen.** (Yes a bed shaker). Use as you would an oven timer. Set the alarm for when your food should come out and when time is up, it will flash, vibrate, and emit a 98-decibel audible alarm; one or any combination will get the attention of someone who is deaf, hard of hearing, or who tends to forget they were cooking.

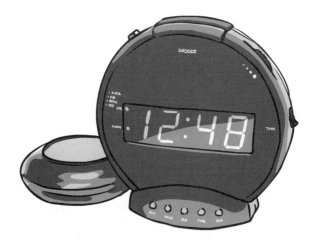

- **Light-weight timers and pagers that are worn on your body** will signal the wearer, by vibration and audible alerts, when it is time to remove dinner from the oven.

174. **Tame electrical cords** either with commercial cord hooks (plastic devices with hooks on each end to keep a cord wrapped), hook and loop fastener tapes, or twisty ties, or by hiding them in empty toilet paper or paper towel tubes.

175. **Wrap pot handles with contrasting tape for better visibility;** always turn pot handles to the inside of the stove.

176. **Remove throw rugs (tripping hazards) and reduce clutter.** A neat and orderly kitchen is safer and much more enjoyable to work in.

RESOURCES

Here are some good resources for making your kitchen more accessible:

Publications by the University of Missouri—Extension

One Handed Kitchen http://extension.missouri.edu/publications/DisplayPub.aspx?P=GH7015

Wheelchair Kitchen http://extension.missouri.edu/publications/DisplayPub.aspx?P=GH5671

Home assessment tools to help you select a variety of kitchen sinks, faucets, and cabinet inserts all in one easy-to-use location, visit www.AdaptMy.com

Aging in Place Video—Kitchen

Aging in Place Professionals

www.aipathome.com—click on Green Mountain Ranch and select "Kitchen"

PRODUCTS

Catalog and Website of Products for Seniors
Aids for Arthritis, Inc.
35 Wakefield Drive
Medford, NJ 08055
Toll free: 800-654-0707
www.AidsforArthritis.com

FirstSTREET
19998 Ruffin Mill Road
Colonial Heights, VA 23834
Toll free : 800-704-1210
www.FirstStreetOnline.com

Appliance Lifts
Dynamic Living—AdaptMy.com
95 West Dudley Town Road
Bloomfield, CT 06002
Toll free: 866-993-0783
www.AdaptMy.com

Kitchen Cabinet Organizers
Kitchen Accessories Unlimited
1136–1146 Stratford Avenue
Stratford, CT 06615
Toll free: 800-667-8721
www.kitchensource.com

Klip! Vibe Mobile Timer
Invisible Clock/Pager
Center for Communication, Hearing, and
Deafness—UniversaLink
10243 W National Avenue
West Allis, WI 53227
Phone: 414-541-5465
Toll free: 800-755-7994
VP toll free: 866-954-9435
TTY: 414-604-7217
www.CCHDWI.org

Learning, Sight, and Sound (LS & S)
145 River Rock Drive
Buffalo, NY 14207
Toll free: 800-468-4789
Toll free TTY: 866-317-8533
www.LSSproducts.com

Plastic Chair Protectors
Home Marketplace
PO Box 3670
Oshkosh, WI 54903
Toll free: 800-356-3876
TTY: 920-231-5506
www.TheHomeMarketplace.com

Shelves That Slide
2050 W Deer Valley Road, Suite F
Phoenix, AZ 85027
Phone: 623-780-2555
Toll free: 800-598-7390
www.shelvesthatslide.com

Slide-Out Dish Storage Cabinet
Kitchen Accessories Unlimited
1136–1146 Stratford Avenue
Stratford, CT 06615
Toll free: 800-667-8721
www.kitchensource.com

Sonic Boom Alarm Clock and Bed Shaker
Center for Communication, Hearing, and
Deafness—UniversaLink
10243 W National Avenue
West Allis, WI 53227
Phone: 414-541-5465
Toll free: 800-755-7994
VP toll free: 866-954-9435
TTY: 414-604-7217
www.CCHDWI.org

Specialty Pans
Walter Drake®
250 City Center
Oshkosh, WI 54906
Toll free: 800-525-9291
www.wdrake.com

Suction Dinnerware
Freedom Distributors, LLC
111 Harris Street
Crystal Springs, MS 39059
Phone: 601-892-3116
www.freedomdinnerware.com

ULU Rocker Knife and Cutting Bowl
Great Northern Products
Anchorage, AK 99516
www.ulu.com
Also available on Amazon.com

Vertical Dish and Pan Organizers
Walter Drake®
250 City Center
Oshkosh, WI 54906
Toll free: 800-525-9291
www.wdrake.com

SEVEN

The Accessible Bathroom

As my physical limitations began to affect my mobility and independence, I couldn't help but think about the future. I could see that before long the bathrooms in our ranch-style house were going to pose some problems. The bathroom in the master bedroom was too small for a wheelchair to get through the door and I didn't want to have to resort to a commode chair. I could still walk a few steps and with the help of my husband Dave, I managed to get to the shower stall where I sat on a lawn chair. But because the shower controls were not within my reach, Dave had to turn the water on and off and redirect the shower head. It was not a perfect situation.

I began to foresee a time when using the bathroom independently would no longer be possible. Remodeling the bathroom seemed to be an option we needed to explore. Everywhere I went—hospitals, clinics, coffee

Accessibility Guidelines

Especially in the bathroom, mere inches make the difference between dependence and independence.

- *Create an unobstructed 60 × 60 inch area in front of the toilet for maximum mobility and maneuverability. Locate the toilet with the centerline 18 inches from a sidewall and allow 24 inches of free space on the other side for safe transfers, mobility devices, and assistance.*
- *To get up and down easier, toilet seats should be 15 to 19 inches high.*
- *Reinforce lower walls (up to 4 feet high) around toilet and bathing fixtures with 3/4-inch plywood to accommodate grab bars.*
- *Widen doorways to 36 inches. Doors should open outward to provide more space inside the bathroom.*
- *A shallow sink mounted 32 to 34 inches high with open knee space underneath will keep the sink within reach of a seated person.*
- *Create a barrier-free shower at least 32 × 60 inches in size with a floor that slopes 2% to a trench drain in the back.*

shops, bookstores, discount department stores—I checked out the bathrooms (the entry, layout, clearances, where grab bars were located, etc.).

Believe it or not, I found my perfect bathroom at Border's Bookstore! Their unisex bathroom was so easy for me to use that I took measurements of everything and applied them to my remodeling plans. Replicating that bathroom improved my safety but more importantly gave me back some of my independence.

If you are in a situation where you're struggling with certain activities and would like some help determining what you need or how to go about setting up or rearranging a room to make it easier for you to manage, visit an Independent Living Center (ILC) a demonstration home, a bathroom design center, or a home health store to try out products and devices that may work for you. Ask your doctor for an assessment by a physical or occupational therapist or a referral to a rehabilitation specialist.

Today, there are thousands of products available to make the bathroom safer and more useable by someone who is getting older or has a disability. The suggestions here merely scratch the surface.

CREATE A BARRIER-FREE FLOOR PLAN

Inches make a big difference in the bathroom. See the Accessibility Guidelines on p. 83 for dimensions to keep in mind.

177. **Give yourself plenty of room to be comfortable**. Generally, you need a 5-foot radius to turn a wheelchair around, so the more room you can create the better.

178. **Widen aisles by getting things off the floor**; get rid of anything that is not necessary—scales, hamper, floor racks, and so on.

179. **Open up closets and cabinets**. Removing doors from closets and replacing cabinets with open shelves, set back from the edge of the countertop, will give you a few extra inches to maneuver while making sinks and storage areas more easily accessible.

180. **For ease of use, the toilet should be located 18 inches from the side wall**, with 2 feet of clear space on the other side to allow for

transfers or assistance. When one side of your body is weaker than the other, use a configuration that feels safer and more comfortable for you.

181. **Entry doors should open to the outside** to give you maximum room to move. If the door opens into a narrow hallway, consider replacing it with a pocket door. To avoid expensive remodeling—tearing out and replacing the wall to mount the door inside—hang the door hardware on the wall outside of the bathroom. To keep a pocket door from sliding all the way into the wall, screw a C-shaped cabinet handle (that your fingers can easily slip into) to the far edge of the door.

182. **If you are unable to reconfigure the bathroom door,** remove it and use a shower curtain rod and shower curtain to give you privacy.

183. **Reduce falling hazards with nonskid tile**. Tile is impervious to water, easy to clean, and easier to move on for the wheelchair user. Nonskid tiles have a special coating that creates a higher friction rate than noncoated tiles. Nonskid coatings are also available to apply to your current flooring; ask about them at your local tile, bath, or home improvement store.

184. **Make the entire bathroom a "wet room."** Consider mounting tile to the walls as well as floors, making the entire bathroom impervious to water. Doing so makes the room easy to clean and maintain.

FAUCETS, SINKS, AND VANITIES

185. **Install a wall-mounted sink**. Not only does it give a sleek, modern appearance to your bathroom but it also maximizes knee-room below the sink. If hot-water pipes are exposed, cover them to protect knees (see Chapter 6 for ideas). If you prefer the look of cabinets, install under-the-counter cabinets that let the basin extend over the edge or hardware that allows doors to slide out of the way when open.

186. **Shallow sink basins are easier to use than a traditional deep sink**. Check out "wading pool" lavatories by Kohler® and

other plumbing manufacturers. Consider installing dual sinks with one at a traditional height and one lower for children or people who need to sit down while grooming.

187. **A pedestal sink stands alone and leaves more room to maneuver**. Keep in mind though that most pedestal sinks do not have counterspace, which may be an issue for folks who need devices or medications as they get ready for the day.

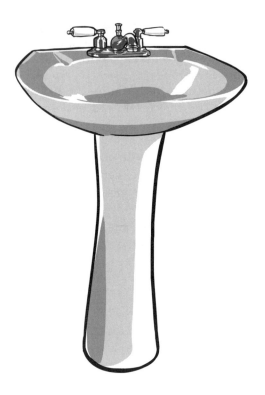

188. **Adjust mirrors to accommodate people of various heights**.

   - **Install a mirror flush to the back splash** so that it is low enough for children or someone who is seated to see themselves.
   - **Tip the top of a wall-mounted mirror a few inches** so that someone who is short or seated can see themselves.
   - **To accommodate multiple heights and abilities, install an adjustable tilt-down mirror**.
   - **An inexpensive alternative is to attach a telescoping mirror**, found in most bath shops, that mounts to the side wall near

the sink, or clamps to or sits on the top of the vanity. Their adjustable, swivel-type necks may easily be moved to various positions. Purchase one with a magnifying mirror on one side to aid those with diminished vision.

189. **Locate the medicine cabinet on the side wall next to the sink** instead of over the sink. This location provides easier access by someone in a wheelchair or with limited arm movement.

190. **Consider installing a kitchen faucet in the bathroom**. Kitchen faucets tend to be longer, reaching further over the sink. When shopping for bathroom faucets, use the closed fist test; if you can operate the faucet with a closed fist, it will be useable by most people, including those with one hand or those with limited grip or reach. Before heading to the bath center, be sure to measure the distance between the handles on your current faucet set.

191. **Consider installing an automatic faucet** or inexpensive sensor that turns the water on when your hand is underneath. Look for these at home improvement stores or order from online stores that cater to the elderly.

TOILETS AND AIDS

192. **Raise the toilet seat**. You will find that raising the toilet seat 4 to 6 inches will make it much easier for you to get on and off the toilet, whether or not you are transferring from a wheelchair. Inexpensive portable seats that fit over your current one are available at drug or home health stores. For a less obtrusive and perhaps more stable lift, raise the whole toilet with a Toilevator® toilet lift.

193. **Install a wall-mounted toilet**. When remodeling or replacing your toilet, consider installing one that is mounted on the wall. Not having a base on the floor reduces tripping hazards, makes it easier to clean around, and gives someone in a wheelchair more room for transferring. (Be sure to consider weight limits before installing.)

194. **Make toileting easier** by adding larger flush handles, long-handled wipe aids, arm supports, or a foot-activated toilet

flusher (available at Amazon.com). A toilet seat in a contrasting color will make it easier to see where to sit.

195. **Install a bidet** that cleanses with water instead of toilet paper. Choose from a state-of-the-art electronic toilet seat with multiple cleansing functions or add a simple personal bidet attachment to your toilet.

TUB AND SHOWER

196. **Create a barrier-free shower area.** Remove any steps or external lips so that you can move easily into or out of the bathing area; zero-threshold shower bases allow you to replace your current shower floor with a fully accessible one.

197. **Slant tile floors toward a trench drain at the back** to make it easier to maintain balance inside the shower. A floor-length, weighted shower curtain will keep water inside or you can install a collapsible water dam that you can easily roll over.

198. **Add a shower seat** that is wall mounted or use a sturdy plastic chair with nonslip feet (available at drug stores), so that you can sit while showering. A padded style with a hole in the middle is more comfortable to sit on and makes hygiene easy.

199. **Exchange your fixed shower head with one on an adjustable bar** or add an inexpensive hand-held shower head with a minimum of a 6-foot hose to your current fixture.

200. **Consider adding a second hand-held shower nozzle in the middle of the long side wall of the shower.** The shower hose coming from the side is easy to use for someone who is seated. An inexpensive solution might be to add a holder for the shower nozzle in this location. *Note*: Make sure standard shower heads and hand-held nozzles work independently of one another and that you can control the water flow on the hand-held.

201. **If a bath is important, consider purchasing a walk-in tub.** Walk-in bathtubs have a door on the side, with a leak-free seal, which lets you simply walk into the tub and sit down on

the built-in seat to bathe. They are expensive but if a soak in a hot tub is what you need, it may be worth the investment. You will find these in catalogs for seniors or at bath remodeling centers. Check with your local home health agency for ideas on funding.

202. **Offset controls in bathtubs and showers**. When remodeling, locate tub and shower controls closer to the outside of tub or shower (rather than in the center of the wall) where it is easy to reach in and set the temperature *before* entering. Raise the controls higher on the wall to minimize bending and stooping or lower for those in a seated position, or install dual controls to accommodate different heights.

203. **Install an antiscald device** and consider a drain that can be operated with your foot; both are readily available at home improvement stores.

204. **In tight spaces, install a toilet–shower seat combination system**. The Wyng® wall-mounted shower system makes it easy to have an accessible toilet and shower in a small space. A hand-held shower is mounted near the toilet which is customized with a special seat, so that your toilet seat becomes your shower seat. This system is expensive but makes it possible to have an accessible shower without removing walls, although you will want to tile the walls and add a trench drain at the back where the floor meets the wall.

205. **Make the edge of the tub easy to see** by draping a contrasting-colored bath mat over the front or by adding a strip of bright-colored tape along the entire top edge. Add a strip of tape to the inside of the tub, too, to indicate the fill line.

206. **Replace standard bathroom washcloths with kitchen cloths, wash mitts** (some come with pockets for the soap), **or net scrubbies**, which are all lighter and easier to grip.

207. **Use soap on a rope in the shower**. Hanging the soap from the shower head or around your neck keeps it within easy reach helping to prevent slips and falls.

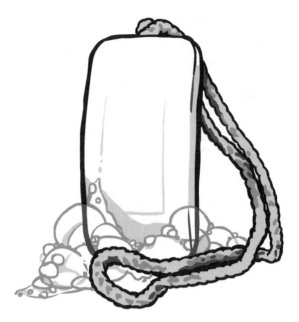

208. **Use long-handled tools,** such as soap holders, brushes, and even hair washers to make it easier to wash without bending or twisting.

209. **Place shampoo, soap, and other bath and body products in brightly colored plastic containers that are easy to differentiate one from the another** and to see against the wall or tub. A rubber band wrapped around the shampoo bottle will distinguish it from the conditioner and make it easier to hold on to.

210. **Use pump-handle containers for shampoo and conditioner** to make them easy for you to use.

211. **Make sure towels are located on a shelf right outside the shower** and robes are on a hook that is easily accessible to the wearer.

212. **Locate your towel storage over a heat vent**, you will have warm towels without additional expense. Electronic towel warmers are another option.

213. **Consider adding heated walls in the shower area** or install a body dryer if you are remodeling your bathroom.

GRAB BARS AND PLACEMENT

Grab bars are essential in the bathroom where humidity and wet surfaces increase the likelihood of slipping and falling. Many styles are available today that are both decorative and supportive, including ergonomically angled and fold-down styles, as well as some that do double duty as towel bars, toilet paper holders, and decorative support built into and around faucets and soap dishes.

214. **Make sure grab bars are installed where they give you the assistance you need**. If you need help determining where the grab bars should be located to provide you with the support you need, consult an occupational therapist or contact your local ILC and ask if they can recommend a builder/remodeler who understands the needs of people with disabilities.

215. **Install permanent grab bars securely** into the studs or a wall reinforced with three-quarter-inch plywood. Only you know the proper height and angle that is right for you. One way to determine where your grab bars should be permanently installed is by trying a portable, suction cup grab bar at various angles and locations.

216. **Install contrasting bars for better visibility**. Install dark bars on light walls, light bars on dark walls, or wrap them with colored tape to make them easier to see. Avoid chrome and other glossy or high-glare finishes.

217. **Consider adding a floor-to-ceiling support pole next to the tub and/or shower**. A variety of support rails are designed for installation over the side of the tub. If these are not secure enough for you, consider installing a transfer pole. For a full description of styles available, see Rails, Lifts, and Other Bedside Aids in Chapter 8, The Accessible Bedroom.

THE LITTLE THINGS

218. **Keep everything you use regularly within easy reach. I have a collection** of clear containers on my bathroom counter that hold cotton balls and other morning necessities; a teaspoon in my toothbrush holder for taking medication; a magnet inside my medicine cabinet to hold my fingernail file; hooks under the sink for my washcloth and hand towel; and my underwear in

a drawer so that it's handy when I get out of the shower. Add a pull-out vanity and use drawer organizers to keep little things where you can find them easily. Organize earrings and other small items in your drawers with a collection of small boxes and ice cube trays held together with binder clips.

219. **Use pump-style containers for lotions and liquid soap.** Liquid soap is easier to handle than bulky bars. Put the soap in a pretty pump-style container and your soap is always at your fingertips. You may want to consider mounting an automatic liquid soap dispenser to the wall.

220. **If you have difficulty blow drying your own hair, try a countertop hair-dryer stand** (available at Target.com). With a stable base and moveable neck, you can easily insert your blow dryer handle into the cushioned holder at the top and by turning your head, dry your hair hands-free, without having to grip or tire your arms. You may find this arrangement helpful in drying hands too.

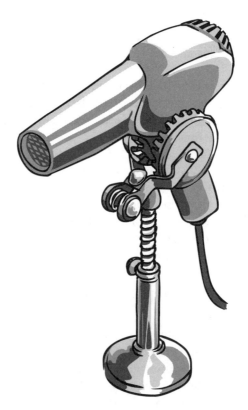

221. **If you have trouble brushing your teeth because of tremors or spasticity, try an electric toothbrush**. The larger handle is easy to grasp and the weight of the toothbrush may improve your coordination, making brushing easier.

222. **Use an electric razor, especially if you have tremors**. An electric razor will shave your skin without the risk of cuts and nicks. Be sure to test how they feel in your hand before purchasing. Or, nix shaving altogether with electrolysis.

SAFETY

223. **Install lighting that provides good visibility when using the sink, toilet, and tub or shower**. Water-tight lighting fixtures for inside shower areas are available at home improvement stores. Don't forget a nightlight so that you can find your way to the bathroom in the dark.

224. **Add additional electrical outlets** to accommodate today's technology and future medical devices; make sure they are water and shock resistant. Unplug electrical devices when not in use and never use electrical devices near a filled sink or tub.

225. **To prevent falls, use a rubberized nonslip bath mat inside *and* outside the tub**. Place a contrasting-colored textured mat inside the tub that will give you a clue to the depth. Make sure any rugs or mats outside the tub are nonslip and contrast with the floor.

226. **Sit down while bathing or showering**. If lifting your leg over the side of the tub is an issue, look for a bath seat that is long enough to put two legs in the tub and two outside so that you can sit down on the seat outside the tub and slide yourself into the bathing area. Make sure the seat legs are adjustable to allow for differences in height between the floor and the bottom of the tub.

227. **Wear a waterproof emergency alert**. Most accidents in the home occur in the bathroom. Be prepared should you slip and fall by wearing a personal alert pendant. Companies like Guardian and Lifeline provide these services. If you have a security system, they may also provide a wearable pendant as a bonus.

Not all companies offer waterproof pendants so be sure to ask if you can take the pendant into the tub or shower with you.

228. **The FreedomAlert® is a programmable, two-way voice communication pendant** that lets you contact up to four relatives, neighbors, or friends, or 911, at the touch of a button. Unlike services, there are no contracts or monthly fees.

RESOURCES

Accessible Bathroom Plans
Residential Rehabilitation, Remodeling, and Universal Design
The Center for Universal Design
College of Design
North Carolina State University
Campus Box 8613
Raleigh, NC 27695-8613
Phone: 919-513-0825
http://www.ncsu.edu/www/ncsu/design/sod5/cud/index.htm

Aging in Place Video—Bathroom
Aging in Place Professionals
www.aipathome.com—click on Green Mountain Ranch and select "Bathroom"

Barrier-Free Shower Design Catalog
AKW MediCare
5390 260th St
Wyoming, MN 55092
Toll free: 888-548-3259
www.akw-usa.com

PRODUCTS

Adjustable "Tilt" Bathroom Mirror
www.Sears.com

Advanced Toilet Seat
Necessity Care
2507 Rhodes Avenue
River Grove, IL 60171
Phone: 708-456-0863
www.NecessityCare.com

Automatic Faucet Adapter
Active Forever
10799 N 90th Street
Scottsdale, Arizona 85260
Phone: 480-767-6800
Toll free: 800-377-8033
www.ActiveForever.com

Automatic Soap Dispenser
Dynamic Living
95 West Dudley Town Road
Bloomfield, CT 06002
Toll free: 866-993-0783
www.AdaptMy.com

Collapsible Shower Dam
Dynamic Living
95 West Dudley Town Road
Bloomfield, CT 06002
Toll free: 866-993-0783
www.AdaptMy.com

Ergonomic, Decorative Grab Bars
Great Grabz®
4535 Domestic Avenue, Suite D
Naples, FL 34104
Phone: 239-403-4722
www.GreatGrabz.com

FreedomAlert® Pendant
EmoryDay, LLC
1121 Annapolis Road, #298
Odenton, MD 21113
Phone: 443-296-2480
www.FreedomAlert-911.com

Long-Handled Washing Aids
Life Solutions Plus, Inc.
2850 Willow Street Pike N, Suite D
Willow Street, PA 17584
Toll free: 877-785-8326
www.LifeSolutionsPlus.com

Personal Bidet and Foot Flusher
American Biffy Company
706 Wells Road
Boulder City, NV 89005
Toll free: 877-422-4339
www.Biffy.com

Pull-Out Vanity
Dynamic Living
95 West Dudley Town Road
Bloomfield, CT 06002
Toll free: 866-993-0783
www.AdaptMy.com

Suction Cup Grab Bar
Aids for Arthritis, Inc.
35 Wakefield Drive
Medford, NJ 08055
Phone: 609-654-8631
Toll free: 800-654-0707
www.aidsforarthritis.com

Tornado Body Dryer
Phone: 317-896-1111
www.TornadoBodyDryer.com

Toilevator®
Allegro Medical
Toll free: 800-861-3211
www.AllegroMedical.com

Wading Pool Lavatories
Kohler® Company
www.Kohler.com

Wall-Mounted Toilet
TOTO® Toilets
www.totoUSA.com

Wyng™ Bath System
240 Stony Creek Way
Millerstown, PA 17062
Toll free: 877-896-1111
www.LifeSolutionsPlus.com

Zero-Threshold Shower Base
Delta Faucet Company
www.deltafaucet.com

EIGHT

The Accessible Bedroom

The bedroom is my sanctuary. It's a place I can escape to when the world around me gets too overwhelming and I need a place to "get my brains back together." It's also where I can recharge my batteries and sleep, giving my body a chance to heal. If the kitchen is the hub, then the bedroom is an island of peace and comfort.

Many years ago, I learned that when I wore certain colors, I looked better. Pinks and bluish reds were flattering, while peach and orangey colors made me look washed out and sick. Since I was spending a lot of time in bed, when we needed to repaint and update the bedroom and master bath, I chose colors that flattered me; I reasoned that it made sense to use the walls in my bedroom and bathroom as a backdrop for me. I also bought bed linens and nightgowns in coordinating colors. The difference was amazing—I felt better and visitors seemed to think I looked better too.

Accessibility Guidelines

To accommodate a wheelchair, scooter, or walker:

- *You will need a 5-foot aisle next to the bed to allow for wheelchair or walker access as well as room for assistance whether personal or with the use of a pole or other assistive device.*
- *Doorways should be 32 to 36 inches wide. Consider using pocket doors on closets and adjacent bathrooms.*
- *Keep things, including all drawers and bedside accessories, within reach of a seated person: 24 inches or less reach from the front or side and 12 inches from the floor.*
- *Closet rods should be within 32 to 54 inches from the floor.*

I also arranged a sitting area to the left side of my bed. Turning my head to the left made it easier for me to visit with family and friends.

Before we had remote controls to operate the ceiling fan and light switches, my husband and a friend (who was an electrician), created a fan and light control box for me at the bed. I loved being able to operate the lights and fan independently. Dimmer switches made it easy for me to control the speed of the fan and the intensity of the lights.

On average, we spend a third of our lives sleeping, and when you have a chronic illness, the number of hours you spend in bed increases. Continue reading to find more tips and ideas for improving your comfort and safety in the bedroom.

BEDS AND BEDDING

Let's start with the largest and the most important feature in the bedroom—the bed itself.

229. **A comfortable mattress is important.** No one can tell you what the best mattress is for you. Whether you choose a traditional innerspring, a memory foam or adjustable "sleep number," a water bed, or an organic cotton hypoallergenic mattress, do your research first and ask about a 30-day sleep guarantee, which is a policy where the company will take the mattress back and return your old one if the new one doesn't work for you. Compare and read reviews of different kinds of mattresses at www.consumersearch.com. You might also go to www.WebMD.com; their sleep disorders section contains an article about choosing the perfect mattress.

230. **Natural organic wool provides therapeutic warmth and cushion for sleeping.** Organic wool batten mattresses, mattress toppers, bedding, and pillows are chemical free and hypoallergenic. Their natural fiber cools in the summer and warms in the winter soothing and relaxing sore muscles for those with fibromyalgia, arthritis, and other painful conditions that make it difficult to sleep.

231. **A Mattress Genie**™ **turns almost any mattress into an adjustable bed.** Use the handy remote control to inflate this cushy

wedge to prop you up to the right angle for eating or watching TV, to relieve congestion or acid reflux, or adjust your position without assistance. The device works on mattresses up to 18 inches in height, *except* for waterbeds.

232. **An alternating air pressure mattress helps folks at risk for pressure sores or with circulatory problems.** These devices, which sit on top of your mattress, have air pockets that are powered by a pump that fills alternate chambers with air causing them to rise and fall, eliminating long-term pressure on any body part. ABLEDATA has information about the different models and features available. Consult your physician about whether or not you would benefit from one of these special devices.

233. **Lift heavy comforters and linens off of your feet.** Heavy blankets can be painful or reduce the ability to move in bed. Whether you choose commercial solutions like an adjustable blanket support, create your own lift frame from PVC pipe or other supplies around the house, or use a cardboard box like I did, getting the linens off your feet is helpful for many people.

234. **The right pillow aids sleep.** The days of "one pillow fits all" are long gone. Not only can you choose from soft, medium, firm, and extra firm and various fills from synthetic fibers to down or feathers, foam, and even memory foam (each with their own advantages), now there are different shapes and sizes to help you find comfort for special conditions as well as if you sleep on your back, side, or stomach.

Here are just a few of the specialty pillows available:

235. **A side-sleeper pillow** is thicker and firmer to support your neck in a neutral position while lying on your side. If made of foam, sometimes they will be contoured to give you breathing channels or places to tuck your hands.

236. **A small contoured "neck pillow"** will provide extra support for your neck when you use a softer pillow.

237. **A back-sleeper pillow** is thin often with extra loft or thickness in the bottom third of the pillow to create a cradle for your neck.

238. **If you sleep on your stomach you want a thin pillow** or perhaps no pillow at all for your head, but you still want something under your stomach to support your back; this is where a "body pillow" may come in handy. The Teardrop™ Orthopedic Body Wedge will help you maintain a proper sleeping position; also works for side sleepers.

239. **If you use a Continuous Positive Airway Pressure (C-PAP) machine**, you know how difficult it can be to get comfortable. A specially designed C-PAP pillow is shaped to support your head while allowing room for the machine's hoses.

240. **For back pain, you may want a wedge pillow** to raise your feet or a pillow that straps around your leg to reduce pressure on hips, knees, and spine. The Dual Position Bed Wedge, made of egg crate foam, provides support for sitting up in bed; turn it around and it provides a 30% incline for sleeping.

241. **Cervical support pillows cradle the head and neck** preventing stress and strain and opening up airways to reduce snoring and sleep apnea symptoms.

242. **If you get overheated while you sleep**, bamboo pillows are antibacterial, hypoallergenic, and naturally wick away heat and moisture. A cold pillow will keep your head cool. Slip the thin Chillow® inside the pillowcase with your pillow or put the Chillow on your mattress with your regular pillow over it. Then turn your pillow over every time you want to feel a cooling sensation.

243. **To support your neck**, try rolling up a hand towel, secure the roll with a couple of rubber bands and insert it into your pillowcase along one of the long edges. Adjust the "neck pillow" for comfort. Or, if you prefer, purchase a tube-like pillow, approximately 24 inches long and 3 inches in diameter, and insert it into the pillowcase along the bottom edge of your regular pillow.

244. **When choosing a pillow, lie down and try it before purchasing**. If you cannot lie down, use the wall to simulate a vertical bed to gauge its comfort for you. For more information on

choosing the best pillow, visit www.WebMD.com and search Sleep Disorders/Choosing a Pillow.

245. **Change pillows every year or two to reduce allergens.** Overtime pillows become a repository for molds, dead skin, and dust mites (ugh!). Wash pillows regularly in hot water to reduce allergens and replace them every year or two to assure proper support. Pillows can be expensive. To extend the life of your pillow and prevent dust mites and bed bugs cover them in finely woven, tightly sealed covers designed specifically for that purpose. You will find a whole selection of hypoallergenic bedding at www.allergybuyersclub.com.

246. **Remove the foot board of your bed to avoid injury in case of a fall.** If you need the foot board to serve as a guide or support, wrap it with a thick blanket or quilt to soften sharp corners.

247. **Raise bed height with bed risers.** Raising the bed, like raising the toilet, can make it easy to get in and out (and as a bonus provides extra storage under the bed.) Inexpensive, heavy-duty black plastic cones will raise the bed 3 or 5 inches and support 1400 pounds. Slightly more expensive 3.5-inch solid hardwood risers can be stacked to raise the bed 7 inches. Of course, you could make your own risers by drilling the appropriate sized hole in a block of wood and raise the bed however high you need.

RAILS, LIFTS, AND OTHER BEDSIDE AIDS

248. **Add bedrails for safety and support.** Children's bedding stores sell a temporary rail that slips under the mattress and prevents someone from rolling out of bed. The rail also serves as a support for sitting up and getting out of bed and a holder for a bed caddy to store your glasses, a TV remote, and so on.

249. **Make a bed caddy out of a color-coordinated hand towel—** fold the ends up and stitch pocket sections to hold eyeglasses, tissues, meds, and so on, then hang over the rail or tuck under the mattress to keep essentials within easy reach while you sleep. Commercially made caddies may be found in catalogs

and on websites that cater to the elderly such as AidsforArthritis.com and firstSTREET.com.

250. **Place mats next to the bed to reduce the risk of injury from falls to someone at risk of seizures or after brain surgery.** Camping stores sell foam pads and antifatigue mats are available in office and home improvement stores. Mats can be pushed under the bed during the day when not in use.

251. **Use a bed cane for support getting in and out of bed.** This cushioned adjustable handle on a stable platform leg gives ergonomic support for getting in or out of bed. It comes with a four pocket organizer for your TV remote, glasses, phone, and so on.

252. **Transfer and support poles and rails increase independence.** If you have difficulty sitting up in bed or getting in and out of bed or an easy chair, you may want to consider installing one or more of the following products by HealthCraft:

   - **Advantage Rail**™ is a floor-mounted support that pivots with you as you take small steps. It provides increased stability getting up and going, yet locks in an instant if you lose your balance. This pole adjusts to various heights and has an antimicrobial finish. You may want to add floor mounts in various locations where you need extra support and take the pole with you to use at locations around the house.
   - The **SuperPole**™ is a floor-to-ceiling support system that can be customized with a full range of accessories (trapeze, tray, support bar) as needed. It installs almost anywhere there is a floor and ceiling up to 140 inches in height; special adaptors are available for slanted ceilings.
   - The **Smart-Rail**™, unlike a fixed bedrail, can unlock and pivot outward to give better support for standing, with less reaching or twisting.
   - The **ModRail**™ is a combination of fixed rail and horizontal bar to provide safety while sleeping yet without hindrance in getting out of bed.
   - **A wall- or ceiling-mounted trapeze** with dual-step handholds that assist the user in pulling themselves to a sitting or a standing position.

DRESSING AREAS, CLOSETS, AND ORGANIZATION

253. **A low dresser is recommended for wheelchair users** because the top drawers of higher dressers are not readily accessible. Dressers with two or three side-by-side columns of narrow, lightweight drawers (18″–24″ wide) with single drawer pulls are easier to access than wider drawers that require double-pull handles.

254. **A resting bench is helpful at the end of the bed**, in the dressing area, or wherever it is most comfortable for you to sit down while dressing. Choose one with storage baskets or drawers underneath the seat and you can keep socks, shoes, and other frequently used items within easy reach.

255. **Install closet bars at varying heights**. Higher and lower bars provide flexibility in hanging tops and bottoms or to place clothing within reach of people of different heights and abilities. Closet systems make this easy or a simple garment rack with multiple height rods may be all you need to make a small closet more accessible.

256. **A weighted closet bar that pulls down to access clothing** and then flips up out of the way might be a nice addition to your closet. *Note:* Before you purchase and install one of these, try it out fully loaded with clothing to see if you have the upper-body strength to use it easily.

257. **Electric closet rods, use a motorized control to lower clothing** on upper rods within reach of a short or seated person. They are more expensive than weighted bars but do not require any upper body strength to operate.

258. **A low-cost way to access clothing on an upper rack** is to purchase or make your own garment hook (a pole with a hook on the end) like they use in boutiques.

259. **Lower storage shelves** are more convenient for people with a restricted range of motion.

260. **A raised shoe shelf** provides convenient elevated storage for wheelchair users and for people who have difficulty bending over.

261. **Shelves, racks, baskets, and lightweight plastic drawers can be substituted for hanging space** if this arrangement better meets your storage and accessibility needs.

262. **A tie rack carrousel is a convenient way to store personal accessories** such as neckties, jewelry, or belts in a relatively small area.

263. **Use drawer organizers to keep socks, underwear, and accessories where you can reach them**. Earrings may be contained and easily retrieved in an empty ice-cube tray.

264. **Organize clothing for the ease of selection.**
     - **If you have trouble telling one color from another**, separate clothing into color groups.
     - **You might try placing different colors that can be worn together along one wall** and other colors in another section of the closet.
     - **Hang an entire outfit on one hanger** (including socks and jewelry) to make selecting clothing easier for someone with limited vision or create tactile markers that slip over the hanger to indicate the color of clothing and aid someone to dress themselves.

COMFORT AND SAFETY

265. **Make reading in bed easy with special glasses**. Bed Spectacles have a 90° prism that lets you read, write, or watch TV comfortably while lying flat. NightVision Readers have bright LEDs built into the frame so that you can read in the dark without disturbing anyone else in the room; corrective lenses are available in 1.5 to 3.0 strengths. See the Resource section for where to purchase.

266. **If you find yourself congested when you sleep, it may be time to add an air cleaner to your bedroom.** Choose a true HEPA filter to trap dust, molds, and other microscopic organisms. For a wide selection of air cleaners tested by people with allergies, visit www.allergybuyersclub.com.

267. Consider getting a "white noise" machine if you are a light sleeper. It produces a soft soothing sound like a light breeze or rushing water to relax you and drown out other sounds that might disturb your sleep. Some models offer a choice of sounds, including a heartbeat for babies. Try them all to see which one works best for you. And there is an App for that!

268. **If you have trouble falling asleep, train yourself to slow down and doze off with a NightWave**™. This device projects a soft blue light on your ceiling. Match your breathing to the rise and fall of the light, and you will soon be relaxed and ready for sleep.

269. **Make sure you have adequate light—not too much or too little.** Compact fluorescent lights (CFLs)—either natural daylight or craft lights are bright without glare.

270. **Install a touch- or clap-activated switch** to the lamp by your bedside.

271. **Add a dimmer to your bedside lamp** and turn it to low just before you go to sleep; that way, if you get up in the middle of the night, you can turn on the light without blinding yourself or disturbing others.

272. **Install a time-activated switch to the light switch by the door** which will give you time to get into bed before the light goes out. Some of these switches can be set to go on or off in 1 to 20 minutes and lower the light intensity slowly to give warning that the light is about to go out.

273. **Plug a Handy Switch**™ **wireless control into any electrical outlet, plug a lamp into it, and use the wireless remote control to turn your lamp on and off** from up to 60 feet away. You'll never have to get out of bed to turn out the light again. The transmitter has a built-in nightlight too.

274. **Use a nightlight to avoid stumbling in the dark.** The Guardian Angel light is four lights in one. Plug it into any wall outlet and set it to nightlight mode—automatically going on at dusk and off at dawn—or motion mode and it will go on whenever

someone walks within 12 feet of it. If the power goes out, it instantly comes on; remove it from the holder and it operates as a regular rechargeable flashlight.

275. **The Verilux® Rise and Shine Wake Up Light is an all-in-one device, with a bedside lamp, alarm clock, and sound machine** that gently awakens you. The light, which is balanced to provide relief from seasonal affective disorder (SAD), slowly grows in intensity as if the sun was rising. Use it at the end of the day to slowly decrease in intensity and trigger your body that it is time to sleep. Audible alarms include nature sounds.

276. **A Sonic Boom Alarm Clock with Bed Shaker attaches to a lamp and the bed.** When the alarm goes off your choice of any combination of the light flashing, the bed shaker vibrating, and/or a loud 98-decibel audible alarm will wake you.

277. **Close closet and dresser drawers immediately** and put shoes and slippers away so you don't trip on them. Keep pathways clear of anything (toys, shoes, purses, etc.) that might trip you up or catch on a mobility devise.

PRODUCTS

ABLEDATA
8630 Fenton Street, Suite 930
Silver Spring, MD 20910
Phone: 301-608-8998
Toll free: 800-227-0216
www.abledata.com

Adjustable Blanket Support
Aids for Arthritis, Inc.
35 Wakefield Drive
Medford, NJ 08055
Toll free: 800-654-0707
www.AidsforArthritis.com

Advantage Rail™/**SuperPole**™, **SmartRail**™, **ModRail**™, **and Trapeze**
HealthCraft Products Inc.
2790 Fenton Road
Ottawa, Ontario, Canada
K1T 3T7
Phone: 613-822-1885
Toll free: 888-619-9992
www.HealthCraftProducts.com

Bamboo Pillows
Herrington Catalog
3 Symmes Drive
Londonderry, NH 03053
Toll free: 800-622-5221
www.HerringtonCatalog.com

Bed Cane
Aids for Arthritis, Inc.
35 Wakefield Drive
Medford, NJ 08055
Toll free: 800-654-0707
www.AidsforArthritis.com

Bed Spectacles
LS&S (Learning, Sight, and Sound)
145 River Rock Drive
Buffalo, NY 14207
Toll free: 800-468-4789
TTY toll free: 866-317-8533
www.LSSproducts.com

Black Plastic Bed Risers
Walter Drake®
250 City Center
Oshkosh, WI 54906
Toll free: 800-525-9291
www.wdrake.com

Chillow® **Pillow**
www.chillow.com

C-PAP Pillow
Walter Drake®
250 City Center
Oshkosh, WI 54906
Toll free: 800-525-9291
www.wdrake.com

Guardian Angel 4-Way Nightlight
Herrington Catalog
3 Symmes Drive
Londonderry, NH 03053
Toll free: 800-622-5221
www.HerringtonCatalog.com

Hardwood Bed Risers
Home Marketplace
PO Box 3670
Oshkosh, WI 54903
Toll free: 800-356-3876
TTY: 920-231-5506
www.TheHomeMarketplace.com

Handy Switch™ Remote Control Light Switch
Aids for Arthritis, Inc.
35 Wakefield Drive
Medford, NJ 08055
Toll free: 800-654-0707
www.AidsforArthritis.com

Mattress Genie™
firstSTREET
1998 Ruffin Mill Rd
Colonial Heights, VA 23834
Toll free: 800-704-1210
www.firstSTREETonline.com

NightVision Readers
Herrington Catalog
3 Symmes Drive
Londonderry, NH 03053
Toll free: 800-622-5221
www.HerringtonCatalog.com

NightWave™
firstSTREET
1998 Ruffin Mill Road
Colonial Heights, VA 23834
Toll free: 800-704-1210
www.firstSTREETonline.com

Organic Wool Mattresses and Bedding
Surround Ewe Sleep Systems/Kerry Hills Farm
N1237 Franklin Rd
Oconomowoc, WI 53066
Phone: 920-474-4503
Toll free: 888-WOOL BED (888-966-5233)
www.SurroundEwe.com

Rise and Shine Alarm Clock Lamp
Verilux, Inc.
340 Mad River Park, Suite #1
Waitsfield, VT 05673
Toll free: 800-454-4408
www.Verilux.com

Sleep Machine/White Noise Machine
Aids for Arthritis, Inc.
35 Wakefield Drive
Medford, NJ 08055
Toll free: 800-654-0707
www.AidsforArthritis.com

Specialty Pillows
Aids for Arthritis, Inc.
35 Wakefield Drive
Medford, NJ 08055
Toll free: 800-654-0707
www.AidsforArthritis.com

Sonic Boom Alarm and Bed Shaker
LS&S (Learning, Sight, and Sound)
145 River Rock Drive
Buffalo, NY 14207
Toll free: 800-468-4789
Toll free TTY: 866-317-8533
www.LSSproducts.com

Center for Communication, Hearing & Deafness
UniversaLink
10243 W National Avenue
West Allis, WI 53227
Phone: 414-541-5465
Toll free: 800-755-7994
VP toll free: 866-954-9435
TTY: 414-604-7217
www.CCHDWI.org

Teardrop™ Orthopedic Body Wedge
Enrichments/Sammons Preston
Patterson Medical
PO Box 5071
Bolingbrook, IL 60440-5071
www.sammonspreston.com

NINE

The Accessible Office: Putting Technology to Work for You

For many years, my "office" was a tiny space located in a little alcove off our master bedroom—not the best place to locate your "place of work." Even while I was in bed resting, I could see the desk, computer, file cabinets, and, of course, the mess. Sometimes I thought I could even hear the work calling to me, "Shelley, you need to answer some emails, you need to write …, you need to call …." But unfortunately, there was no other location in our house to carve out another office area.

Since my office was used for work (writing articles and books), I contacted the state Division of Vocational Rehabilitation (DVR) to see if they could assist me. Each state has vocational rehabilitation (VR)

Accessibility Guidelines

To accommodate a wheelchair, scooter, or walker:

- *Allow 5.5 feet between the desk and any other furniture or file cabinet. This will automatically give you the 5-foot turning radius needed for a wheelchair, scooter, or walker.*
- *Doorways should be 32 to 36 inches wide. Consider using folding or pocket doors on closets.*
- *Keep everything, including all file drawers, equipment, and accessories, within reach of a seated person: 24 inches or less reach from the front or side and 12 inches up from the floor.*
- *Closet shelving should be within 12 to 54 inches from the floor.*

services to help people with disabilities prepare for, enter, retain, or regain employment. VR services can also pay for products you need to get a job or to continue working. I applied for, and because of my level of disability, I was able to receive services. The first modification they made for me was a computer keyboard tray for my desk. The tray held the keyboard at a right angle to my desk, which, in my case, made the keyboard easier for me to use.

Today, stores offering office equipment and supplies have hundreds of options and choices for creating an accessible office. So whether you work from home or simply want a space to pay bills, organize household papers, or organize your medical records, here are some ideas you may want to consider. *Note*: These tips may also be helpful in creating an accessible office at your place of employment.

GETTING STARTED

For assistance in determining your needs, ask your doctor for a referral to a physiatrist (a doctor who specializes in physical medicine and rehabilitation) and/or a physical/occupational therapist. These medical professionals can do a full assessment of your limitations and abilities, provide tips for working smarter, and advise and give you valuable information and/or recommendations on products (chairs, desks, computer setup, glasses, repetitive strain programs, etc.).

You can begin your research for office products by consulting the Resources listed at the end of this chapter. Your local Independent Living Center (ILC) has a wealth of knowledge to assist you in determining what will make your life easier, and they often have loan closets where you can try a product before you buy it.

FURNITURE AND PLACEMENT

278. **Create a wrap-around work area** with desk surfaces 24 to 28 inches deep on both sides and front; not only does that configuration put everything you need within reach and give you room to spread out, you will also have support on three sides to help

you to move within the space. One side of the desk might contain drawer storage for files you use regularly; the other might provide a roll-under surface for additional workspace and conferring with visitors.

279. **Consider adding drop-down/lift inserts** into overhead storage shelves or cabinets for books, directories, and supplies that you need within reach but perhaps do not use everyday.

280. **Create multiple work surfaces/heights to match the job.**
     - **To prevent wrist injury**, a keyboard should be 3 to 5 inches lower than the desktop.
     - **A pull-out keyboard tray**, available in most computer desks, gives you a lower level for the keyboard. Pull the tray out to bring the keyboard closer to you; slide it in when you are not using it.
     - **An adjustable keyboard tray** that raises, lowers, and tilts back or forward allows you to set the angle most comfortable for your wrists. These trays, available at Amazon.com and most office supply stores, mount to and fit into the knee-cutout in most computer desks.

281. **Whenever possible, stand up to work.** It has now been proven that standing up to work is healthier than sitting at a desk all day. If you have the option, try it for all or part of your work duties and see if you like it. Use an overturned box to temporarily raise up the work surface to a comfortable height. Make sure you have carpeting or rubber fatigue mats under your feet when you stand for long periods.

282. **Allow 5.5 feet between desk and files and any other furniture** (chair, sofa, file cabinets, side table, credenza, etc.) in the room. This will allow adequate space for a wheelchair or walker user to get around easily. And be sure to keep floors and aisles free of clutter.

283. **Optimize ergonomics.** If you sit most of the day, be sure that your body is supported properly.

284. **Get a chair that conforms to you.** Look for one with an adjustable height so that your feet rest comfortably on the floor

(additional back and seat adjustments are nice also), short armrests that support your arms, and padded support for your lower back (lumbar) and thighs. Sit in the chair at the store before you purchase it. If you are of smaller stature, a "secretarial chair" with arm supports may be better than an executive chair that is made to fit the average male.

285. **A number of ergonomic devices (adjustable keyboard trays, arm supports, etc.) are made to customize work areas.** Ask about what is available at an office design center or consult a rehabilitation specialist, such as an occupational therapist.

286. **If you are working, ask your employer or vocational rehabilitation agency for a free ergonomic assessment by a qualified rehabilitation specialist** or ask your physician for a referral to a physiatrist or physical/occupational therapist.

287. **Make sure you stop work and get up and move around regularly.** If you need a reminder, there are computer programs like Google's "Take a Break" that will prompt you to do so.

288. **Enhance your ability to hear clearly.**
    - **Carpet and draperies muffle sharp sounds,** making it easier to hear.
    - **Position chairs where you can easily see a person's face and they can see yours.** If you have a hearing impairment, maximize your ability to understand what is being said by sitting with your back to a window. The light from the window will illuminate the faces of those who you are speaking with and you'll be able to see their lip movements and facial expressions to help you follow what's being said.
    - **Looping systems enhance the hearing ability of people who wear hearing aids.** This technology, which only works with telecoil hearing aids, can enhance hearing in a small area or a whole room.
    - **If you have a mild hearing loss, consider using a personal sound amplifier** and/or hearing aids.

TECHNOLOGY

Computers

Computers have removed barriers in our world in ways we couldn't have imagined even 5 years ago. Today, just by sitting in front of a computer, we can shop for hundreds of products to make our homes safer and more user friendly, do research on services and resources for making our lives easier, and communicate with home accessibility experts anywhere in the world.

289. **Before you buy a computer, go to a computer store with "experts"** who can explain what kinds of computers are currently on the market (laptop, tablet, desktop, etc.). To assess your needs and abilities and make recommendations for you personally, consult a rehabilitation technology specialist through your hospital or clinic rehabilitation department. If you need a computer for work, consult with your state's Vocational Rehabilitation agency; they will often do a free assessment and provide the equipment and accessories you need.

290. **All computers have accessibility features built into their operating system** (PC or Mac) that let you slow down the blinking speed of the cursor, convert two simultaneous keystrokes to two consecutive keystrokes, convert text to speech or speech to text, and more. Consult your User's Guide or Help function to find out more about the accessibility features of your computer. You might also consider taking a class to learn how to get the maximum benefit out of your computer.

Vision Aids

If you are losing your vision due to age, illness, or macular degeneration, it can be a confusing and frightening time. There are many products that can enhance your vision and make it possible to "see" what you are doing.

291. **Computer technology now makes it possible to have text translated to sound.**

292. **Contact the National Council of State Agencies for the Blind** to find an office in your state that can refer you to local service organizations.

293. **Ask your eye specialist to refer you to a therapist who can do an assessment** and make recommendations for your specific situation.

TELEPHONES AND OTHER COMMUNICATION AIDS

Today, there are all kinds of telephones to keep us connected. However, if you cannot hold the handset, see clearly enough to dial the number, or hear what the caller is saying, contact your local telephone company's special-needs department. They may sell adaptive telephone equipment and provide services, such as free directory assistance and operator-assisted dialing to their customers with special needs.

294. **Speaker phones let you talk on the phone while leaving your hands free.** Whether it makes it easier to take notes or is just more comfortable for those with arthritis, weak grip, or other hand challenges, a speaker phone is a great way to conserve energy when using the phone. If dialing is also an issue, look into voice-activated and programmable models.

295. **Large button and photo dialer phones are easy to use for people with poor manual dexterity or low vision.** Serene Innovations® has a series of amplified phones with large easy-to-see buttons as well as photo dialing for those with limited hearing and vision.

296. **Amplified phones enhance speech tones while muffling background noise** so that you can hear the caller better. Some add-on devices allow you to amplify incoming call volume without buying a new phone.

297. **Captioned phones show what the caller is saying.** A digital read-out screen on the phone shows the incoming conversation in text format so that you can read and confirm that you heard correctly. These phones require using a telephone relay system for the Deaf that uses voice recognition software to translate words to text. You will also need an Internet connection.

298. **TTY text telephones use a keyboard to type the conversation.** TTYs use a relay service operator who translates the typed message from the deaf person and reads it to the hearing person. Then, it takes the hearing person's response and types the message for the deaf person to read.

299. **Video phones let the Deaf talk with friends or family using sign language.** These phones provide high-definition video over a high-speed Internet connection.

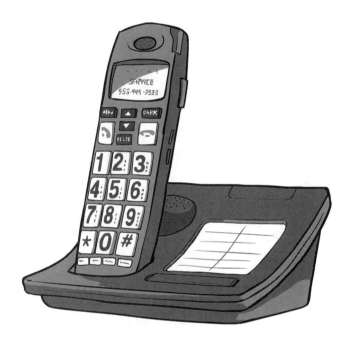

To find out more about the above telephone and communications devices, see the Resources section of the end of this chapter.

300. **Fund telecommunications equipment purchases with Telecommunications Equipment Purchase Program (TEPP).** People with disabilities may qualify for TEPP funding to purchase telephones, TTYs, video phones, and other telephone-related equipment. Every state handles this program differently, so contact your county social services agency or ILC and ask about TEPP funding.

301. **Smartphones put the power of the Internet at your fingertips.** In addition to sending and receiving phone calls, smartphones

offer text messaging for the Deaf, voice recognition for dialing numbers or doing Internet searches for those with physical or visual impairments, screen magnification, turn-by-turn navigation, and many other helpful features. Check with local cellular providers for models and features available. Be sure to ask about service plan discounts for the Deaf and other people with disabilities.

302. **VoIP (Voice-over Internet Protocol) services like Skype™ let you see and hear the caller.** This is nice for "face-to-face" meetings and communicating with family a long distance away. Since calls are made through your computer and require an Internet connection, there are no telephone long-distance charges. However, because Internet speeds vary, this technology may not have high-enough definition for the Deaf to use for sign language.

303. **Voice amplification devices boost speech volume.** If you have a weak voice due to Parkinson's disease, MS, surgery, or another larynx condition, some amplified phones can increase your outgoing call volume as well as incoming. For everyday communication, the ChatterVox® boosts a weak voice with a microphone worn near the mouth connected to a small speaker and power supply worn around the waist.

ORGANIZING AND SAFETY

304. **Keep chargers and portable electronic devices (phones, DPAs, etc.) corralled with a charging station.** Charging stations are available in the gift section in department stores or where office supplies are sold. Create your own recharge station by slipping a power strip into a shoe box; plug all the chargers into the strip. Cut Xs in the top of the box for each charger wire; slip the end that connects to the device through the hole, tying the excess wire with a twist tie; be sure to mark the end of each wire with the name of the device the cord belongs to. When you come home or go to bed at night, plug the device into the charger; the box top will provide a shelf. In the morning, unplug and go. To conserve energy, be sure to turn the power strip off in the morning or when not charging.

305. **Use a digital recorder to take notes or make a grocery or errands list.** Some recorders combine with speech-to-text programs to automatically enter your notes into your computer.

306. **Lateral files are easier to use by most people.** Because of their height, they are easily accessible by people in wheelchairs and offer an additional work space or a place for printers, scanners, and other devices that is easy to reach from a seated position. To find files easier, color code them.

307. **Get rid of wires—go wireless.** As you purchase new office equipment, consider getting wireless-enabled products that can talk to each other. Not only will the lack of wires look nicer, but without wires you reduce a potential tripping hazard.

308. **If wireless is not an option, contain the wires as follows:**
    - **Tie groups of wires with twisty ties** to keep them together.
    - **Use colored rip-and-stick cable wraps** to help you identify which wire is which; red might be for the main computer, blue for the printer, and so forth. Another option is to wrap a file label around each cable to identify which device it operates.
    - **Add a row of stick-on hooks to the back of your desk;** run the cords through and bundle them with twist ties. This will keep them off the floor and out of the way.

309. **Add dimmer switches** so you can adjust the light up or down as needed.

310. **Install task lighting where you need it.** Goose-neck or architect-style lamps can be adjusted easily to put the light where you need it.

311. **Install hands-free switches on lights and lamps,** either motion or sound activated.

312. **Allow for natural light wherever possible;** use automatic blinds to control natural light levels.

RESOURCES

ABLEDATA provides objective information about assistive technology devices. www.abledata.com

Accessible Devices is a company that offers a wealth of information on assistive technology for people with disabilities, including email updates and podcasts. To learn about the many assistive devices, visit www.accessible-devices.com.

e-Bility.com features Web links on accessibility subjects. Look to them for information, resources, services, and products of interest to people with disabilities and those who love and care for them.

Microsoft Accessibility Resource Centers are located in most states of the United States and around the world. The staff will show you how to use accessibility features and how to select assistive technology products that are right for you. If you do not live near a center, a link to an online Assistive Technology Decision Tree will help you determine which products might work best for your particular impairment. (*Note*: The document looks a bit daunting at first, but just answer the questions, "Yes" or "No" and follow the arrows to the appropriate product selections.) You may wish to print this document and take it with you to your state's Vocational Rehabilitation agency or an ILC for assistance in further determining and obtaining the proper equipment for your needs. Here is the link to the Assistive Technology section of the Microsoft Website: http://www.microsoft.com/enable/at/types.aspx.

The National Multiple Sclerosis Society has a large resource section on assistive technology. Visit www.NationalMSSociety.org and search on Assistive Technology.

The Abledbody website (www.abledbody.com) has emerged as a trusted voice on disability issues to consumers, businesses, and the media. They cover assistive devices and technologies.

Technology Assistance Act Program. Depending on your disability and financial need, you may qualify for help from the federal Technology Assistance Act Program. Contact your county social services agency for the office that administers this program in your state.

The Center for Communication, Hearing, and Deafness
10243 W National Avenue
West Allis, WI 53227
Phone: 414-541-5465
Toll free: 800-755-7994
VP toll free: 866-954-9435
TTY: 414-604-7217
www.CCHDWI.org

National Council on Independent Living
1710 Rhode Island Avenue Northwest
Fifth Floor
Washington, DC 20036
Phone: 202-207-0334
Toll free: 877-525-3400
TTY 202-207-0340

National Council of State Agencies for the Blind
www.ncsab.org

PRODUCTS

ChatterVox®
39 Crestland Road
Indian Creek, IL 60061
Phone: 847-816-8580
www.Chattervox.com

Drop-Down/Lift-Up Cabinet Inserts
Dynamic Living/AdaptMy.com
95 West Dudley Town Road
Bloomfield, CT 06002
Toll free: 866-993-0783
www.AdaptMy.com

In-Line Phone Amplifier
LS&S (Learning, Sight, and Sound)
145 River Rock Drive
Buffalo, NY 14207
Toll free: 800-468-4789
www.LSSproducts.com

Looping Systems
Center for Communication, Hearing, and Deafness
10243 W National Avenue
West Allis, WI 53227
Phone: 414-541-5465
Toll free: 800-755-7994
VP toll free: 866-954-9435
TTY: 414-604-7217
www.CCHDWI.org

Personal Sound Amplifier
Center for Communication, Hearing, and Deafness
10243 W National Avenue
West Allis, WI 53227
Phone: 414-541-5465
Toll free: 800-755-7994
VP toll free: 866-954-9435
TTY: 414-604-7217
www.CCHDWI.org

Where You Can Learn More

Included below are just a few of the thousands of resources providing information for people with disabilities. Learn more online or at your local library.

ALL DISABILITIES

ABLEDATA A source for assistive technology and product information.
8630 Fenton Street, Suite 930
Silver Spring, MD 20910
Phone: 301-608-8998
Toll free: 800-227-0216
www.abledata.com

National Library Service for the Blind and Physically Handicapped A national service that provides Braille and talking books, newspapers, and publications for people with disabilities.
Library of Congress
Washington, DC 20542
Phone: 202-707-5100
Toll free: 888-NLS-READ (888-657-7323) which connects to your local library
TTY: 202-707-0744
www.loc.gov/nls

National Rehabilitation Information Center (NARIC) Home to more than 70,000 resources (books, reports, articles, and audiovisual materials), relating to disability and rehabilitation research, and includes databases of agencies and organizations, directories, journals and other periodicals, and online resources.

8201 Corporate Drive, Suite 600
Landover, MD 20785
Phone: 301-459-5900
Toll free: 800-346-2742
TTY 301-459-5984
www.naric.com

RESOURCES FOR PEOPLE COPING WITH CHRONIC ILLNESS, DISABILITY, OR AGING

AARP   A resource for people over 50.
601 E Street, NW
Washington, DC 20049
Toll free: 888-OUR-AARP (888-687-2277)
Toll free TTY: 877-434-7598
www.aarp.org

Adaptive Devices and Independent Living Aids
Patterson Medical/Sammons Preston (Distributor of general and
    medical products for a wide variety of disabilities.)
1000 Remington Boulevard, Suite 210
Bolingbrook, IL 60440-5117
Toll free: 800-323-5547
www.pattersonmedical.com

Assistance Dog United Campaign
1221 Sebastopol Rd
Santa Rosa, CA 95407
Phone: 707-545-0800
www.AssistanceDogUnitedCampaign.org

Disabilities Resources Monthly   A guide to disability resources on
    the Internet.
Disability Resources, Inc.
Dept. IN
4 Glatter Lane
Centereach, NY 11720-1032
Phone: 631-585-0290
www.disabilityresources.org

Making Life Easier—The Newsletter   Solutions in the form of tips,
    products, and strategies for living for people with chronic illness,
    disability, or age-related limitations.

Meeting Life's Challenges, LLC
The home of Tips for Making Life Easier
9042 Aspen Grove Lane
Madison, WI 53717-2700
Phone: 608-824-0402
www.MeetingLifesChallenges.com
www.MakingLifeEasier.com

The Complete Directory for People With Disabilities   A comprehensive directory and reference book you might ask your library to purchase for you and others in the community.
Grey House Publishing
PO Box 56
Amenia, NY 12501-0056
Phone: 518-789-8700
Toll free: 800-562-2139
www.greyhouse.com/disabilities.htm

RESOURCES FOR THE BLIND AND THOSE WITH LOW VISION

American Council of the Blind and Visually Impaired
2200 Wilson Boulevard, Suite 650
Arlington, VA 22201
Phone: 202-467-5081
Toll free: 800-424-866
www.acb.org

American Foundation for the Blind
2 Penn Plaza, Suite 1102
New York, NY 10021
Phone: 212-502-7600
Toll free: 800-AFB-LINE (800-232-5463)
www.afb.org

Lighthouse International
The Sol and Lillian Goldman Building
111 East 59th St
New York, NY 10022-1202
Toll free: 800-829-0500
www.lighthouse.org

National Association of State Agencies for the Blind   Directory of contacts by state.
www.ncsab.org

National Council of Private Agencies for the Blind and Visually Impaired   A comprehensive list of resource links for the blind and visually impaired.
8760 Manchester Road
St. Louis, MO 63144
Phone: 314-961-8235
www.agenciesfortheblind.org

Talking Books and Braille Services

National Library Service for the Blind and Physically Handicapped
Library of Congress
Washington, DC 20542
Phone: 202-707-5100
Toll free: 888-NLS-READ (888-657-7323) which connects to your local library
TTY: 202-707-0744
www.loc.gov/nls

HARD OF HEARING AND DEAF RESOURCES

American Speech-Language-Hearing Association
2200 Research Boulevard
Rockville, MD 20850-3289
Phone: 301-296-5700
Toll free: 800-638-8255
www.asha.org

National Institute on Deafness and Other Communication Disorders
National Institutes of Health
31 Center Drive, MSC 2320
Bethesda, MD 20892-2320
Toll free: 800-241-1044
Toll free TTY: 800-241-1055
www.nidcd.nih.gov

OTHER DISABILITY RESOURCES

Attainment Company, Inc. Products for people with speech and
language impairments.
504 Commerce Parkway
PO Box 930160
Verona, WI 53593-0160
Toll free: 800-327-4269
www.attainmentcompany.com

Environmental Working Group Information on and advocacy for
nontoxic living.
1436 U Street, NW, Suite 100
Washington, DC 20009
Phone: 202-667-6982
www.ewg.org

National Alliance for Caregiving
4720 Montgomery Lane, 2nd Floor
Bethesda, MD 20814
www.caregiving.org
www.familycaregiving101.org

National Alliance on Mental Illness
3803 N Fairfax Drive, Suite 100
Arlington, VA 22203
Phone: 703-524-7600
Toll free: 800-950-NAMI (6264)
www.nami.org

Nearly every chronic illness and disability has a support group (or
groups) dedicated to the issues and challenges of that condition.
Contact your local library for contact info for a support group
near you.

READING LIST

Some of these are oldies but goodies. Look for these and other publications at your local library. If they do not have them, perhaps they
will order them for you.

A Consumer's Guide to Home Adaptation
Institute for Human Centered Design
200 Portland Street
Boston, MA 02114
Adaptive Environments, 2002
Phone/TTY: 617-695-1225
www.adaptenv.org

Accessible Home Design: Architectural Solutions for the Wheelchair User
Thomas D. Davies, AIA and Kim Beasley, AIA
PVA Distribution Center
Paralyzed Veterans of America, 2006
Toll free: 888-860-7244
www.pva.org

Building for a Lifetime: The Design and Construction of Fully Accessible Homes
Margaret Wylde and Adrian Baron-Robbins
Taunton Press, 1994
63 S Main Street
PO Box 5560
Newtown, CT 06470-5506
Phone: 203-426-8171
Toll free: 800-477-8727
www.taunton.com

Easy Things to Make to Make Things Easy
Doreen Greenstein
Brookline Books, 1997
Cambridge, MA

Eighty-Eight Easy-to-Make Aids for Older People and for Special Needs
Don Caston
Hartley & Marks, 1988
Point Roberts, WA

Living a Healthy Life With Chronic Conditions
Kate Lorig, RN, DrPH, Halsted Holman, MD, David Sobel, MD, Diana Laurent, MPH, Virginia Gonzalez, MPH, and Marian Minor, RPT, PhD
Bull Publishing Company, 2007
Boulder, CO

Living With Low Vision: A Resource Guide for People With Sight Loss
Resources for Rehabilitation, 1996
Lexington, MA
22 Bonad Road
Winchester, MA 01890
Phone: 781-368-9080
www.rfr.org

Making Life More Livable: Simple Adaptations for Living at Home After Vision Loss
Maureen A. Duffy
AFB Press, 2002
American Foundation for the Blind
2 Penn Plaza, Suite 1102
New York, NY 10021
Phone: 212-502-7600
Toll free: 800-AFB-LINE (800-232-5463)
www.afb.org

Index